Vaccine Hesitancy Curriculum

Amanda J. Chase • Michelle L. Demory
Marc M. Kesselman
Editors

Vaccine Hesitancy Curriculum

A Guide for Health Professions Educators

Springer

Editors
Amanda J. Chase
Department of Medical Education,
Dr. Kiran C. Patel College of Allopathic Medicine
Nova Southeastern University
Fort Lauderdale, FL, USA

Michelle L. Demory
Department of Medical Education,
Dr. Kiran C. Patel College of Allopathic Medicine
Nova Southeastern University
Fort Lauderdale, FL, USA

Marc M. Kesselman
Chair, Department of Internal Medicine,
Chief Division of Rheumatology,
Dr. Kiran C. Patel College of Osteopathic Medicine, Nova Southeastern University
Fort Lauderdale, FL, USA

ISBN 978-3-031-88667-6   ISBN 978-3-031-88668-3 (eBook)
https://doi.org/10.1007/978-3-031-88668-3

This Springer imprint is published by the registered company Springer Nature Switzerland AG
The registered company address is: Gewerbestrasse 11, 6330 Cham, Switzerland

Preface

Vaccination can be considered one of the greatest triumphs in promoting human health, beginning in the eighteenth century with the smallpox vaccine. While early skepticism of vaccines was widespread, modern science and medicine established vaccination as a cornerstone of the standard of care. For generations, vaccination was considered one of the surest ways to prevent death and suffering from infectious diseases. However, with advances in social networking and the rise of an anti-vaccination movement, vaccine hesitancy is once again a problem facing healthcare providers. The importance of mitigating health misinformation by training healthcare providers to communicate with patients and the community about vaccination is paramount. For clinicians and practitioners to have empathetic and productive conversations with patients, it is important to understand the spectrum of hesitancy, informed by patient motivations and medical historical events.

This book provides a historical view of vaccine hesitancy in addition to a novel repository of approaches to cultivate communication skills, deliberate practice, and reflection in health professions trainees. The COVID-19 pandemic reignited the importance of mitigating health misinformation and mistrust in vaccines by training health providers to communicate with patients and the community about vaccination. To understand patient perceptions of vaccination, this book takes a deep dive into the rationales behind vaccine apathy, hesitancy, and resistance. Additionally, this book provides resources on how to effectively communicate various topics that center around the delivery, function, adverse effects, and research of vaccines.

The first few chapters of this book focus on understanding the origins of vaccine hesitancy, reviewing landmark events that ignited mistrust of vaccination, and examining the range of factors that surround vaccination resistance. With any type of resistance, there is a spectrum of opinions and perceptions within the community, these can range from vaccine hesitancy to conspiracy. Clinicians need to quickly assess where their patients fall on this spectrum and to pivot their approach and communication strategy accordingly. Moreover, it is important for clinicians to understand the importance of historical, cultural, and societal elements influencing vaccination decisions. With this understanding, effective strategies can be applied to clinical practice.

Subsequent chapters present approaches to integrate vaccine education into health professions curricula and cultivate communication skills in health professions trainees. The educational literature informs us that systemic curricular modifications, with longitudinal threads that incorporate vaccine education, are more effective than single sessions in educating health professions learners and clinicians on how to approach vaccine hesitant patients. When applied to patient care, vaccine conversations have the power to counteract vaccine misinformation, dispel myths, and engender trust, particularly in vulnerable populations. The final chapter serves as a source of clinical cases and facilitator notes for promoting the acquisition of communication skills that will help learners to effectively communicate with patients and protect vulnerable communities from misinformation. When implemented into health professions education, these communication strategies prepare future clinicians with the knowledge, skills, and attitudes necessary to identify, prevent, and challenge mistrust in science and vaccines.

Our hope is that this book will serve as a driver for transformative change in a way that will positively impact learning in health professions education and contribute to a critical appraisal of the impact of vaccine hesitancy and mistrust on patients and communities. We thank every contributing author, many of whom tapped into their own personal and professional experiences to construct the content presented in this publication.

Fort Lauderdale, FL, USA Amanda J. Chase
Fort Lauderdale, FL, USA Michelle L. Demory
Fort Lauderdale, FL, USA Marc M. Kesselman

Contents

Chapter 1
A History of Vaccine Hesitancy

Stephanie Nagy, Michael Wu, and Marc M. Kesselman

Globally, vaccination campaigns historically have been the most significant and successful public health interventions. Vaccines are a crucial tool in preventing and limiting the spread of life-threatening diseases, as four million deaths each year are prevented as a result of childhood vaccinations [1]. However, there has been a decline in vaccination rates, in 2021 only 81% of infants received their full vaccine coverage, the lowest in over a decade, and there are over 18 million children who have received zero doses of their childhood vaccinations, the highest since 2005 [2]. Vaccination exemption rates increased in 41 states, with over a 5% exemption rate in 10 states in 2023 [2]. The significant reductions in vaccination status can be largely attributable to vaccine hesitancy, previously referred to as vaccine resistance or vaccine opposition [3]. Vaccine hesitancy is defined by the Strategic Advisory Group of Experts Vaccine Hesitancy Working Group of the World Health Organization as the intentional delay or refusal of vaccination when vaccines are readily available and accessible [4]. It has been described as one of the top 10 threats to public health in 2019 and continues to be a prevalent risk [4]. The hesitation surrounding vaccinations has been predominant since the first vaccine was created against the deadliest disease at the time, smallpox. Vaccinations were a crucial tool in the fight against smallpox, leading to the first-ever eradication of a widespread disease in 1980 [5]. Vaccine hesitancy is a complex issue that varies across history and is context-specific; however, its incidence continues to be widespread. In this chapter, we will explore the historical events that continued vaccine hesitancy

S. Nagy · M. Wu
Dr. Kiran C. Patel College of Osteopathic Medicine, Nova Southeastern University, Fort Lauderdale, FL, USA

M. M. Kesselman (✉)
Department of Internal Medicine, Chief Division of Rheumatology, Dr. Kiran C. Patel College of Osteopathic Medicine, Nova Southeastern University, Fort Lauderdale, FL, USA
e-mail: mkesselman@nova.edu

A. J. Chase et al. (eds.), *Vaccine Hesitancy Curriculum*,
https://doi.org/10.1007/978-3-031-88668-3_1

among specific populations, the history surrounding the misinformation of common vaccines, and the topic of adverse reactions vs. allergies to vaccines.

1.1 Confidence, Complacency, and Convenience: The Key to Overcome Vaccine Hesitancy?

Many factors play a role in the development of vaccine hesitation, in 2011, the "3 Cs" model was developed by the World Health Organization EURO Vaccine Communications Working Group to understand better the vaccine hesitancy determinants [6]. The "3Cs" of "confidence," "complacency," and "convenience" were determined to be the leading factors that can impact the hesitation one has for vaccinations. Confidence is defined as the trust in the effectiveness and safety of the vaccine, the healthcare system and professionals providing the vaccine, and the motives of policymakers. Vaccine complacency refers to an individual's perception of certain vaccine-preventable diseases as being low risk to their health and, as a result, not deeming the vaccine necessary for their well-being. Finally, convenience is crucial in the appeal of vaccine uptake, including the affordability, geographical accessibility, and health education available [6]. The "3Cs" are a critical framework to follow in the production of vaccination campaigns to ensure tailored, educational, accessible, and culturally competent campaigns to boost confidence and compliance and provide convenience for all to receive the vaccine.

1.2 Historical Events Leading to Mistrust of the Healthcare System by Racial Groups in the Present Day

Outside of the concerns pointing at the safety and efficacy of specific vaccines, another crucial barrier against vaccinations is the medical mistrust between certain racial groups as a result of historical wrongdoings by the healthcare system. The impacts of these events are passed down through generations, continuing to promote medical mistrust with healthcare providers, leading to increased vaccine hesitancy and skepticism.

The Tuskegee syphilis study is cited as one of the most significant catalysts for the mistrust minority populations, specifically African Americans, feel with the healthcare system. The Tuskegee syphilis study began in 1932 by the United States Public Health Service recruited 600 African American males, 400 with syphilis and 200 without, in Macon County, Alabama, to analyze the natural progress of syphilis; however, subjects were not informed of this true research goal [7]. Participants were told they would be receiving treatments for "bad blood," which at the time referred to a variety of conditions, including anemia, syphilis, and fatigue, and incentivized them with free health testing, fresh meals, and the covering of funeral expenses, but they received no treatment at all [7]. At the time of the initiation of the study, no treatment for syphilis had yet be discovered until 1947, when penicillin had been found to be the treatment of choice; however, the researchers withheld the life-saving medication in order to continue the study without informing participants [7]. The study continued until 1972, 40 years after its initiation, due to public knowledge of the study and outcry for its termination. From 1932 to 1972, dozens of African American males involved in the study died from syphilis, and it also led to the spread of syphilis due to the lack of effective treatment even when one was identified 30 years prior to the conclusion of the trial [7]. Amid the Tuskegee study, throughout the twentieth century until the late 1970s, numerous state-sponsored sterilization programs were opened, resulting in the sterilization of 65,000 Americans based on the new science of the time, "eugenics" [8, 9]. Eugenics was the thought process that American society would prosper and succeed if only made up of Anglo-Saxon and Nordic people who were white and non-disabled, which led to all other minority groups being seen as unfit for society. This thought process resulted in African American, Hispanic, and Indigenous men and women and also those with disabilities being forcefully sterilized; however, women were sterilized at a substantially higher rate [8]. For example, in California, between 1920 and 1945, Latina women were at a 59% greater risk of forced sterilization than white women. African American women also made up 43% of the women sterilized in federally-funded family planning programs, while they only made up a third of the population [10]. The unlawful, widespread coerced sterilization of minority groups in the twentieth century has since been deemed a human rights infringement, but its effects continue to be seen.

The historical wrongdoings of the medical field against minorities continue to be a significant barrier for ethnic groups to receive adequate and proper healthcare, including vaccinations, due to the lack of trust in the medical system [11, 12]. Medical mistrust is a significant factor limiting vaccine uptake. The greater the mistrust, the lower the odds of vaccination intent or obtainment [13]. The perception of healthcare providers being deceiving or misinformed by minority groups continues to trickle down as research of harmful studies like the Tuskegee study and the widespread forced sterilization of minority women.

1.3 Analyzation of Misinformation and Common Myths Surrounding Modern-Day Vaccinations

The anti-vaccination movement dates back to 1796 when Dr. Edward Jenner discovered the first vaccine in England for smallpox prior to the major modern-day vaccination campaigns for the smallpox vaccine in the 1950s [14]. Dr. Jenner received opposition from clergy members and physicians regarding the safety and effectiveness of this novel prevention method [15]. The shift away from textbooks and physical medical journals reserved for medical personnel to the accessibility of medical information to the public through the press of a button on the internet has shifted the physician–patient dynamic. Patients are able to play a larger role in the decision-making process due to more information in layman's terms; however, the internet also lends itself to disseminating false and misleading information that can hinder a patient's health. Anti-vaccination campaigns are readily accessible and are often the first results patients find when searching the internet. Davies et al. found when conducting a Google search of the terms "vaccination" or "immunization," 43% of the results were anti-vaccination campaigns in addition, YouTube videos opposing vaccines had higher ratings and views than pro-vaccine videos even though they only made up 32% of the videos on vaccinations [16]. Additionally, it was found that 43% of social media posts containing health-related misinformation were regarding vaccines [17]. With the growth of social media being a key distribution channel for the public to receive information without verification of the reliability and quality of the information, it has been a widely exploited channel for misinformation. Anti-vaccination campaigns and speculation continue to be crucial in building up the hesitation patients may have with vaccines, and many use the past speed bumps in vaccinations as proof for their cause.

Below, we will explore the history of common modern-day vaccines, the misinformation and bias surrounding them, and the resulting impact of it.

1.4 Live Vaccines

Live vaccines were the first form of vaccine subtypes to be discovered. Live vaccines consist of the attenuated form of the virus to mimic a response similar to a weakened natural infection in the body to promote a strong antibody and cellular response leading to long-lasting immunity. Live vaccines are considered more effective than their counterparts of killed vaccines that require additional doses to obtain a similar immune status to live vaccines after a singular dose. However, concerns surrounding live vaccines are geared toward reversing the virus to full virulence, resulting in a more severe infection, and are not recommended for pregnant or immunocompromised [18, 19].

1.4.1 Smallpox

Smallpox is a part of the poxvirus family, which is transmitted through respiratory droplets that have sloughed off of oropharyngeal lesions, leading to the aerosolization of the particles or through direct contact with active open lesions that have not crusted over. Smallpox infection occurs within 3–4 days of exposure and disseminates to the bone marrow, spleen, and lymph nodes, with a secondary viremia occurring 8–12 days later, causing the virus to enter the oropharyngeal mucosa and small vessels. The symptomatic presentation of smallpox initially begins with fever, headache, chills, and abdominal pain with skin lesions that can spread to all areas of the body, most commonly the extremities and face. The skin lesions are often described as round, firm, deep-seated, and well-circumscribed and transition between the phases of macules to papules to vesicles to pustules and finally to crusts, where they become noninfective [20–22].

Taking a look back into the history of smallpox is crucial to understanding the rush to find a prevention or cure for this rapidly infectious disease. The smallpox virus spread throughout the Middle Ages and was introduced to the New World by conquistadors. The smallpox virus quickly spread throughout the army during the Revolutionary War, from 1775 to 1781. The Revolutionaries were not only fighting against one another but also the smallpox virus. It is said that for every soldier who was killed in battle, the smallpox virus killed 10 [23]. The mortality rate was 180 per 1000 soldiers. During the seven years of the Revolutionary War, 63,000 soldiers died as a direct cause of smallpox infection; however, only 7000 died due to direct combat [24, 25]. Smallpox crippled the army and raised the urgency to develop a successful prevention method against it. At first, inoculation was trailed to prevent the extent of infections in soldiers. Inoculation included the process of removing pus from active smallpox lesions and placing it under the skin of noninfected patients with a similar goal to our modern-day vaccines to induce a milder form of the infection to build an immune response if the body comes in contact with the fully-active form of the virus. However, it carries high risks of converting into fully active disease states and disseminating around the body, leading to further spread in communities [14]. Dr. Edward Jenner, known as the "Father of Vaccinations," created the first modern-day vaccine in 1797 by utilizing the cowpox virus, a harmless strain of the smallpox virus. He discovered that infecting a person with the cowpox virus provided immunity against smallpox [14]. The method of vaccination consisted of inoculating the pustular material from a smallpox lesion from one individual to the other in a manual scratch made on the patient's arm, which was then replaced by the modern method of utilizing heat-stable freeze-dried injectable vaccine, which now allowed for widespread vaccination campaigns leading to the eradication of the virus in the 1980s. However, even with the profound impacts the smallpox vaccine has made in removing the deadly virus from modern-day society, at the time, Dr. Jenner faced hashed criticism by physicians and clergy members of the church in regards to the safety of the vaccine and moral basis surrounding infecting patients with a virus [14]. In the 1870s and 1880s, anti-vaccination campaigns began to spread throughout Europe, resulting in significant declines in the smallpox vaccine uptake, in Stockholm, Sweden the rates of vaccination dropped from 90% to 40%; however, after an outbreak, the vaccination rates rose [26, 27]. The smallpox vaccine was crucial in eradicating one of the deadliest diseases in human history and was the sole reason the virus was deemed eradicated in the 1980s after widespread vaccination campaigns using the modern-day form.

Since its declared eradication in the 1980s, routine vaccinations against smallpox have been discontinued. However, two major vaccines are FDA approved for smallpox: ACAM2000 and JYNNEOS (also called Imvamune or Imvanex) for high-risk populations. AMCAM2000 is a single-dose vaccine containing the vaccinia virus, which also belongs to the poxvirus family; however, it is a less infective virus compared but still leads to effective prevention against smallpox. Common side effects of Imvamune include rash, fever, and head and body aches. It is recommended as a routine vaccination for those in constant direct contact with any orthopoxviral, including the replication-competent vaccinia virus, which can cause human infections. For healthcare professionals, Imvamune is not recommended as a routine vaccination; however, it is available as required. JYNNEOS is a replication-deficient live vaccine administered in two doses in 4-week increments for individuals who have never been vaccinated against smallpox before or one dose for those who have received a previous smallpox vaccine [28].

1.4.2 Measles–Mumps–Rubella Vaccine

The Measles–Mumps–Rubella (MMR) is a combined vaccine to prevent all three diseases. Measles is a member of the Paramyxoviridae family; it is commonly spread through inhalation of exposed infective droplets that initially infect the recipient's lymphocytes, dendritic cells, and alveolar cells found in the respiratory tract, which then has the capability of hematogenous spread to distant organs [29]. Measles belongs to the Paramyxoviridae family, with primary replication occurring in the respiratory tract, specifically within the upper airway mucosal epithelium, before spreading to regional lymph nodes. The most common presentation is parotitis, characterized by unilateral swelling of the parotid gland, which may lead to severe permanent effects of deafness [30, 31]. Rubella is a part of the Matonaviridae family, which is spread through respiratory droplets and replicates in the nasopharyngeal cells and regional lymph nodes with hematogenous dissemination. Often a maculopapular rash is seen on the face and neck initially, then spreading to the torso and limbs. Rubella is particularly significant to prevent, as it can spread through vertical transmission from mother to infant, potentially leading to miscarriages or congenital malformations, known as congenital rubella syndrome (CRS). CRS includes cataracts, deafness, congenital heart disease, and dermal erythropoiesis, commonly termed "blueberry muffin" [32, 33].

The MMR vaccine was developed as a combination vaccine in 1971, given in two doses, between 12 to 15 months and 4 to 6 years. It has been found to be very effective as a preventive measure against these three viruses. Currently, two vaccines are approved: M-M-R II and PRIORIX. They are interchangeable, and each contains live and attenuated versions of all three viruses [31, 34]. After the first dose, there was 90% prevention against rubella, and after the second dose, there was 99% and 95% prevention against measles and mumps, respectively. Additionally, the vaccine has been found effective as a post-exposure treatment to measles, reducing the severity of the illness in specific populations, such as individuals who are severely immunodeficient, recent recipients of a bone marrow transplant, those treated for acute lymphoblastic leukemia, and individuals infected with HIV [34].

The effectiveness of the MMR vaccine was overshadowed in 1998 by Dr. Wakefield and colleagues' publication in *The Lancet*, which indicated the link between the MMR vaccine and neuropsychiatric dysfunctions such as autism in children. The study that took place in the United Kingdom consisted of 12 children and claimed that the onset of behavior abnormalities, including loss of acquired skills and communication abilities, occurred after receiving the vaccination [35]. However, the paper's findings were never replicated by other researchers, and the paper was retracted in 2010 by all authors except Dr. Wakefield, who maintained his belief in this link. *The Lancet* additionally conducted its investigation into the findings of the study and concluded that the 12 children were carefully chosen, medical records for each subject could not be reproduced that matched the descriptions and diagnoses, and the funding of the project was provided by lawyers representing families conducting lawsuits against vaccine companies [36, 37]. Many researchers tried to replicate these findings; however, none found any connection between the MMR vaccine received and the onset of autism [38–41]. Nonetheless, the findings of the paper spread like wildfire throughout the world, concerning parents and caregivers not only the MMR vaccine but the safety and efficacy of all vaccines. Following the article by Dr. Wakefield, vaccination rates fell from 88% to 80% in the United Kingdom five years after the publication, and the country has continued to recover in MMR vaccination [42]. The publication of this study not only tarnished the public's view on the effectiveness of the MMR vaccine but also left a long-standing negative impact across all vaccines leading to speculation and mistrust.

1.4.3 Poliomyelitis Vaccine

The poliovirus (Polio) belongs to the Picornaviridae family that is transmitted mainly through the fecal-oral route, leading to replication within the oropharynx, lymphoid tissues, and the gastrointestinal tract. The majority of patients exposed to poliovirus are asymptomatic; common symptoms can present as gastroenteritis, respiratory tract infections, and influenza-like symptoms [43]. However, poliovirus can also transmit and replicate within the central nervous system, leading to paralytic polio. Patients with paralytic polio may develop paresthesia, muscle pain, loss of superficial and deep reflexes, difficulty swallowing, and, in severe cases, paralysis [44]. In the 1900s, polio began to spread rapidly, prompting the WHO to launch the Global Polio Eradication Initiative. With the help of vaccines, the initiative successfully eradicated all three wild forms of poliovirus by 2002 in the majority of the world. By 2021, polio remained endemic only in Pakistan and Afghanistan [45]. The Global Polio Eradication campaign would not have been possible without the production of the inactivated polio vaccine and the oral polio vaccine. Dr. Jonas Salk pioneered the first inactivated polio vaccine in 1955, and the oral form was created in 1961 by Dr. Albert Sabin [45].

The development of polio vaccinations was a crucial milestone leading to its 99.99% eradication worldwide; however, the start of the polio vaccine experienced a few setbacks in its early production. The Cutter Incident in 1955 negatively tarnished the public's view on the safety of the processing of vaccines after active forms of the polio virus were included in the vaccine instead of the inactivated vaccine due to missteps taken at the Cutter Laboratories. This incident led to 120,000 doses containing the live polio vaccine to be given to children, resulting in 56 developing paralytic poliomyelitis and 5 deaths in addition to 100,000 additional contacts, of which 113 developed paralysis and 5 additional deaths in close contacts from those originally infected [46, 47]. Additionally, from 1955 to 1963, 10–30% of polio vaccines were administered with simian virus 40 (SV 40). It is estimated that 98 million Americans received these contaminated vaccines, which were produced using monkey kidney cell cultures to grow the poliovirus. At the time, SV40 was being investigated as a teratogen in animals, causing mesothelioma, osteosarcoma, ependymoma, and lymphomas [48]. Since then, polio vaccines have been SV 40 free, and no correlation has yet been found between humans and the development of cancer [49–52]. However, despite the oversight that resulted in the Cutter Incident and the addition of SV 40 to cultures, it led to the development of more stringent regulations and systems to ensure the safety in the processing of vaccines to prevent another similar occurrence.

1.5 Inactivated Vaccines

Inactivated vaccines contain a version of the virus that has been altered to destroy its disease-producing capability. Unlike live vaccines, inactivated vaccines cannot regain their infectious properties. However, they tend to produce a weaker immunological response, often requiring subsequent immunizations to achieve adequate coverage [53].

1.5.1 Diphtheria–Tetanus–Pertussis (DTP) Vaccine

The Diphtheria–Tetanus–Pertussis (DTP) vaccine is a combined vaccine aimed at the prevention of all three diseases. Diphtheria is a respiratory disease caused by toxigenic strains of corynebacterial diphtheria [54]. This toxigenic strain is contracted via respiratory droplets and has been linked to respiratory illness as well as possible cardiac and neurologic complications. Tetanus is a respiratory and musculoskeletal disease caused by spore-forming clostridium tetani [54]. Tetanus is contracted by inoculation of spores through nonintact skin that can lead to painful contractions of the jaw and muscles with possible progression to respiratory failure [54]. Pertussis is a respiratory disease caused by the bacteria *Bordetella pertussis*. The disease is contracted via respiratory droplets and is known to cause an intense spasmodic cough that can lead to vomiting and a characteristic inspiratory whoop. Vaccines combating these diseases were originally created as monovalent vaccines aimed at preventing a singular antigen. The whole-cell pertussis vaccine was created in the 1920s but was not recommended for children until the 1940s. In 1991, a less reactogenic acellular vaccine was introduced with quicker induction of usage in children [54]. The tetanus vaccine was discovered in 1924 after the discovery of tetanus toxin inactivation with formaldehyde in the early 1920s [55]. The tetanus toxoid vaccine gained popularity with widespread usage in World War 1. The diphtheria toxoid vaccine was created in the early 1920s and was not widely adopted until the 1930s [56].

The DTaP combination vaccine was first introduced in the 1940s after the advancement of universal vaccination in efforts to combat diphtheria, tetanus, and pertussis [57]. The vaccine combines diphtheria, tetanus toxoid, and the acellular pertussis antigen. The vaccine aims to generate an active immune response in the body with the creation of antibodies and antitoxins against the toxoids and acellular pertussis antigens. There are currently two FDA-approved combination vaccines approved for usage in the United States. They are recommended to be dosed at 2 months, 4 months, 6 months, 15–18 months, and 4–6 years. Most adverse events are associated with specific antigens within the vaccine. The whole-cell pertussis vaccine has been linked to local adverse effects such as redness, swelling, and pain. The tetanus toxoid has been linked to brachial neuritis, but this has been studied and is extremely rare [57]. The National Childhood Encephalopathy Study investigated the causal relationship between DTP and nervous system dysfunctions and claimed that the DTap vaccine resulted in permanent brain damage due to the risk of febrile seizures in the first 24 h. However, follow-up studies have been unable to confirm this finding, and children who did experience febrile convulsions in the first 24 hours had no long-term effects on follow-up studies [58]. Some concern has been raised regarding administering the DTaP vaccine with other vaccines, but the CDC's Advisory Committee on Immunization Practices (ACIP) has advised the coadministration of vaccines with the DTaP to be a safe practice [57].

1.5.2 Human Papillomavirus Vaccine

Human papillomavirus (HPV) is a naked DNA virus that replicates in the stratified squamous epithelia and is known to cause numerous clinical presentations via various strains of the infectious virus. HPV is one of the most commonly sexually transmitted diseases, with virus transmission being through sexual skin contact. HPV has been found to have over 40 different virulent strains, with other most common presentations known by patients and physicians are anogenital warts and respiratory papillomatosis being caused by HPV strains 6/8 and cervical cancer being caused by HPV 16/18. An estimated 630,000 cases of cancer have been attributed to HPV, with an estimated 35,000 cases of cancer caused by HPV each year in the United States [59].

Vaccine development aimed to prevent cancer by combating the highly oncogenic HPV-16 and HPV-18 strains. The HPV vaccine is composed of self-assembled virus-like particles that form when microbial organisms produce an HPV protein through the fermentation process [60]. The HPV virus-like particles act as an antigen that provokes the body to produce HPV-neutralizing antibodies. To date, there are only two vaccines aimed at combating HPV. The bivalent Cervarix vaccine is aimed at combating HPV-16 and HPV-18, and the Gardasil Quadrivalent vaccine is aimed at treating HPV-6, HPV-11, HPV16, and HPV-18. The Gardasil vaccine is the only vaccine that is FDA-approved in the United States at this time. The Federal Advisory Committee on Immunization Practices (ACIP) and the American College of Obstetricians and Gynecologists (ACOG) have endorsed the usage of the vaccination. The vaccination has been recommended for all women between the ages 9–26 and is administered in three doses at the first dose, then 2 months later and 6 months later [60].

There have been concerns around the HPV vaccine but many of them have been dispelled as this vaccine has been proven to be safe and effective. One concern is the vaccine causing ovarian failure; this has been squandered as this effect is only seen in 1 in 10,000 women. In a study of 200,000 women, only 46 had ovarian failure, and none of the cases could be linked back to the vaccination [61]. Another concern has been the usage of the vaccine could be linked to autoimmune disease or death. Studies have been conducted in population groups ranging from hundreds to millions of people, and none of the studies have found a linkage between the vaccine and autoimmune disease or death. The last concern is that the vaccine is unsafe and has not been tested enough. Clinical vaccine testing has been conducted numerous times, demonstrating an excellent safety profile each time. The ACIP found that in clinical trials with tens of thousands of people, patients were just as likely to have acute injection reactions as participants receiving the placebo vaccine. They also found in their trials that the vaccine participants had rates of autoimmune disease similar to those of placebo patients. Finally, post-approval surveillance through the Vaccine Adverse Events Reporting System (VAERS) and Vaccine Safety Datalink (VSD) has only found a risk of syncope after vaccine administration. In a study of over 600,000 HPV vaccine doses, the only identified symptom was syncope, as confirmed by the VAERS and VSD. VAERS and VSD have also found no linkage to death or autoimmune disease with vaccine usage in post-approval surveillance [61].

1.6 mRNA Vaccines

mRNA vaccines are the newest form of vaccination, receiving its first FDA approval in 2020 against severe acute respiratory syndrome coronavirus 2 (SARS-CoV-2), also known as COVID-19. Investigation into the use of mRNA as a foundation for vaccines began in the 1970s. The mRNA vaccine is a synthetically formulated fragment of a specific RNA sequence of the virus, which triggers the body's immune response to create antibodies, which then allows the immune system to have a faster and stronger effect against the true form of the virus [62].

1.6.1 COVID Vaccine

The SARS-CoV-2 is a highly infectious positive-sense, single-stranded RNA virus that spreads via droplet respiratory droplets. The virus contains an S-protein that allows attachment and entry into the host cell and has served as a vaccine target (Chung). The virus's rapid spread is responsible for the worldwide pandemic beginning in March 2020. Between March 2020 and March 2022, 480,905,839 confirmed cases of COVID-19 worldwide and 6,123,493 patient deaths due to virus or other complications have been recorded [63]. Some of the common signs and symptoms associated with the virus are muscle aches, headaches, sore throat, and diarrhea. Some variants of the virus have been identified, such as Alpha, Beta, Gamma, Delta, and recently identified Omicron. A few new variants of interest have also emerged, such as Lambda and Mu. The emergence of the new variants has contributed to the need for a vaccine able to combat the new variants as the variants have presented with a mutation in the spike protein, threatening the efficacy of the COVID-19 vaccine [64, 65].

The COVID-19 vaccine is a mRNA vaccine that has been developed and FDA-approved for intramuscular injection in efforts to combat COVID-19. The vaccines utilize an mRNA sequence that encodes the COVID-19 S-protein, which is surrounded by a lipid nanoparticle for stability [66]. Once injected, the mRNA is translated into the COVID-19 spike protein, which activates T-cells in the body, leading to B-cell activation and subsequent antibody production against the COVID-19 spike protein. The antibodies created by the body allow for both neutralization and destruction of the virus upon infection. The bivalent Moderna and Pfizer vaccines are the only two vaccines the FDA has approved for injection. The Moderna vaccine is dosed twice with the second dose delivered 28 days after the initial dosage. In a study of 30,000 patients by Mascellino et al., the Moderna vaccine demonstrated an efficacy of 94.5% against COVID-19 disease and 100% efficacy against severe disease [66]. The Pfizer vaccine is also dosed twice, with the second dose delivered 21 days after the initial dose. A study of 43,000 patients conducted by Mascellino et al. found that the vaccine efficacy against disease corresponded to 95%, and the efficacy against severe disease corresponded to 87.5% [66].

Fear of the COVID-19 virus has become widespread after its emergence and emergency usage authorization by the FDA. Many of these concerns are rooted in myths and misinformation but have gained traction and become the beliefs of many. A major concern to the public was how quickly these new form of mRNA vaccines was produced and available for distribution, and they questioned the research behind them and their safety. However, mRNA vaccine research and production were not a new concept as since the 1970s, pharmaceutical companies have investigated the use of mRNA as potential vaccines, and from 2005 to 2016, it was discovered the use of lipid nanoparticles as an outer envelope can help deliver the mRNA to cells. Investigation into mRNA vaccine was already on the go when the COVID-19 pandemic began, and from the start of the pandemic, companies already began looking for a cure, which allowed them to quickly distribute the vaccines after FDA approval [67, 68]. After mass COVID-19 vaccination campaigns began, one of these myths is that the mRNA vaccine alters the DNA in the person injected. This has been dispelled as tests have shown the mRNA does not enter the nucleus and is broken down by various RNAases [69]. Myocarditis has also been of concern in patients after receiving the COVID-19 vaccination. Rosner et al. conducted a study where they found 7 patients with myocarditis after Pfizer vaccine administration found resolution of all symptoms and suggested that the risk–benefit decision for vaccination remains highly favorable [70]. Another concern has been central venous thrombosis in patients after vaccine administration. In a study of four million people, it was found that possibly five cases of central venous thrombosis had been reported with multiple factors involved in the pathogenesis of this disease, not solely due to vaccine administration [63]. The COVID-19 vaccine has been subject to many myths and implicated as a possible cause of various extremely rare adverse effects, but the vaccine has been demonstrated to be safe and effective against the COVID-19 virus and its devastating effects.

1.7 Concerns Regarding Vaccine Safety: Adverse Reactions vs. Allergies

Adverse reactions and allergic reactions after vaccination delivery have frightened parents and clinicians for years. The severity and signs and symptoms vary based on the event that is taking place after the vaccine administration. By definition, any event linked directly to vaccine administration after delivery is an adverse reaction [71]. These reactions can range from local effects, such as redness and swelling at the injection site, to systemic reactions, such as body aches and fatigue [71]. Although most of these events resolve independently and may require no medical assistance, the event can worsen into a serious adverse event. A serious adverse event is when an undesirable experience is associated with using a medical product on a patient [72].

Allergic reactions fall under the category of adverse reactions but differ from the previously discussed local and systemic reactions [71]. Allergic reactions are, by definition, idiosyncratic reactions that are caused by an immunologic mechanism [73]. The reactions are broken up into two categories: immediate and delayed types of reactions. These reactions occur due to hypersensitivity to either a vaccine antigen or a different vaccine component [73]. Providers should be vigilant of patients with allergy history as they may be at increased risk for allergic reactions upon vaccine administration.

Some adverse events due to vaccine additives have gained popularity and have led to vaccine hesitancy recently. A few of the vaccine adjuvants that have led to this hesitancy are thimerosal, formaldehyde, monosodium glutamate, polysorbate 80, and various metals. Thiomersal has been used as an adjuvant in vaccines and is hypothesized to be linked to autism. In a study by Parker et al., they evaluated 12 research papers that have drawn an association between autism and thimerosal [74]. Through their study, they concluded that there was no linkage between the two, and studies that found linkage had flawed designs that rendered the conclusions invalid. Formaldehyde has been used in vaccines as an agent to detoxify various bacterial toxins. Although formaldehyde is a carcinogen, the dosage found in vaccines is about tenfold less than what is found in normal human circulation [75]. The usage of aluminum salts as vaccine adjuvants has gained attention as harmful to the human body through neurotoxicity even though, to date, no studies have found a link between vaccine administration and metal toxicity [76]. No population-based studies regarding aluminum and vaccines have been conducted, but billions of vaccines have been administered to individuals around the world, with no linkage between aluminum in vaccines and neurotoxicity being identified [77]. It is clear to see why parents have hesitancy when subjecting their children to vaccine administration. However, research into the topic displays evidence, so it is clear to see that these vaccine adjuvants have been studied and are safe.

Aside from the various vaccine adjuvants, some additives have been linked to common allergens such as eggs, yeast, and gelatin. Egg hypersensitivity has been found to have a prevalence in up to 1.7% of the population, with 70% of people outgrow the allergy by age 16 [78]. Some of the vaccines containing egg products that have worried parents are the influenza vaccine, MMR, rabies, and yellow fever vaccines [79]. Of the four vaccines, influenza has been the vaccine to present the biggest problem to those with egg allergies, and many clinicians have given the vaccine with great caution to those with egg allergies. Recent findings have shown that the risk of anaphylaxis due to vaccine administration is extremely low and does not warrant skin testing anymore [80]. Gelatin is added as a stabilizer in various vaccines, such as MMR, Varicella, and DTaP [81]. Individuals with a gelatin allergy have been found to have reactions to these vaccines. If an allergy exists or is suspected, it is recommended to slowly administer the vaccine in incremental doses under supervision. Individuals who do not have an allergy are safe from all vaccinations with gelatin stabilizers. Yeast has also been an additive of interest in vaccines such as the Hepatitis B vaccine. According to VAERS, 107 adverse events were reported in individuals with a yeast allergy, and 11 of those were possible allergic reactions to the Hepatitis B vaccine. The vaccine has demonstrated safety, but those with a pre-existing or suspected yeast allergy should be given the vaccine in incremental doses and under supervision [81].

Vaccines are a source of modern medicine that has aided in the prevention of countless diseases and advanced the health of many. With these advances, though, comes the associated fears of adverse events and allergic reactions to vaccines. Through research, it is clear that some of the fear linked to adverse events has been minimized and dispelled. Steps have also been taken to minimize the effects and possibilities of allergic reactions in those with allergies and receiving vaccinations.

1.8 Conclusion

Vaccines have been a significant milestone in Public Health's initiative to prevent and spread deadly illnesses across the globe. With the development of this life-changing technology, it is inadvertent that they will be met with hesitation from the general public. However, since their inoculation, vaccines have consistently shown their effectiveness and general safety in preventing diseases that often had a high mortality rate prior to vaccinations. Vaccine hesitancy may continue to be prevalent as with any health advances; however, the importance of proper health education and disputing misinformation is critical to reducing misconceptions and reluctance among the general public.

References

1. Centers for Disease Control and Prevention. (2024). Fast facts on global immunization. https://www.cdc.gov/global-immunization/fast-facts/index.html
2. Seither R, Yusuf O, Dramann D, Calhoun K, Mugerwa-Kasujja A, Knighton A. Coverage with selected vaccines and exemption from school vaccine requirements among children in kindergarten—United States, 2022–23 school year. Morb Mortal Wkly Rep. 2023;72(45):1217–24. https://doi.org/10.15585/mmwr.mm7245a2.
3. Kumar D, Chandra R, Mathur M, Samdariya S, Kapoor N. Vaccine hesitancy: understanding better to address better. Isr J Health Policy Res. 2016;5(2) https://doi.org/10.1186/s13584-016-0062-y.
4. World Health Organization. (2019). Ten threats to global health in 2019. https://www.who.int/news-room/spotlight/ten-threats-to-global-health-in-2019
5. Gallegos M, Pecanna V, Caycho-Rodriguez. Anti-vax: the history of a scientific problem. J Public Health. 2022; https://doi.org/10.1093/pubmed/fdac048.
6. MacDonald N, SAGE Working Group on Vaccine Hesitancy. Vaccine hesitancy: definition, scope and determinants. Vaccine. 2015;33(34):4161–4. https://doi.org/10.1016/j.vaccine.2015.04.036.
7. Centers for Disease Control and Prevention. (2024). About the untreated syphilis study at Tuskegee. https://www.cdc.gov/tuskegee/about/index.html
8. Kluchin RM. Fit to be tied: sterilization and reproductive rights in America, 1950–1980. Rutgers University Press; 2009.
9. Dowbiggin IR. Keeping America sane: psychiatry and eugenics in the United States and Canada, 1880–1940. Cornell University Press; 2018.
10. Novak NL, Lira N, O'Connor KE, Harlow SD, Kardia S, Stern AM. Disproportionate sterilization of Latinos under California's eugenic sterilization program, 1920–1945. Am J Public Health. 2018;108(5):611–3. https://doi.org/10.2105/AJPH.2018.304369.
11. Thomas M, Amstutz C, Horter J, Holben D. Medical mistrust among food insecure individuals in Appalachia. J Health Promot Maint. 2023;46(3):192–202. https://doi.org/10.1097/FCH.0000000000000362.

12. Prall S, Scelza B, Davis HE. Medical mistrust, discrimination and healthcare experiences in a rural Namibian community. Glob Public Health. 2023;19(1) https://doi.org/10.1080/17441692.2024.2346207.
13. Allen J, Fu Q, Shrestha S, Nguyen K, Stopka T, Cuevas A, Corlin L. Medical mistrust, discrimination, and COVID-19 vaccine behaviors among a national sample U.S. adults. SSM Popul Health. 2022; https://doi.org/10.1016/j.ssmph.2022.101278.
14. Riedel S. Edward Jenner and the history of smallpox and vaccination. Baylor Univ Med Cent Proc. 2005;18(1):21–5. https://doi.org/10.1080/08998280.2005.11928028.
15. Raja N, Jothy A. Edward Jenner's discovery of vaccination: impact and legacy. Cureus. 2024;16(9) https://doi.org/10.7759/cureus.68993.
16. Keelan J, Pavri-Garcia V, Tomlinson G. YouTube as a source of information on immunization: a content analysis. JAMA. 2007;208(21):2481–4. https://doi.org/10.1001/jama.298.21.2482.
17. Suarez-Lledo V, Alvarez-Galvez J. Prevalence of health misinformation on social media: systematic review. J Med Internet Res. 2021;23(1) https://doi.org/10.2196/17187.
18. Ginglen JG, Doyle MQ. Immunization. StatsPearls Publishing; 2023.
19. Yawetz S. Patient education: vaccination during pregnancy (beyond the basics). UpToDate; 2023. https://www.uptodate.com/contents/vaccination-during-pregnancy-beyond-the-basics/print
20. Breman JG, Henderson DA. Diagnosis and management of smallpox. N Engl J Med. 2002;346(17):1300–8. https://doi.org/10.1056/nejmra020025.
21. Moore ZS, Seward JF, Lane JM. Smallpox. Lancet. 2006;367:425–35. https://doi.org/10.1016/s0140-6736(06)68143-9.
22. Milton DK. What was the primary mode of smallpox transmission? Implications for biodefense. Front Cell Infect Microbiol. 2012;2:150. https://doi.org/10.3389/fcimb.2012.00150.
23. Beckler A. Smallpox in Washington's army: strategic implications of the disease during the American revolutionary war. J Mil Hist. 2004;68(2):381–430. https://www.jstor.org/stable/3397473?origin=JSTOR-pdf
24. Liebowitz D. Smallpox vaccination: an early start of modern medicine in America. JCHIMP. 2017;7(1):61–3. https://doi.org/10.1080/20009666.2016.1273611.
25. Stanhope BJ. The evolution of preventive medicine in the United States Army, 1607–1939. Office of the Surgeon General Department of the Army; 1968. https://apps.dtic.mil/sti/pdfs/ADA291762.pdf
26. Nuwarda R, Ramzan I, Weekes L, Kayser V. Vaccine hesitancy: contemporary issues and historical background. Vaccine. 2022;10(10):1595. https://doi.org/10.3390/vaccines10101595.
27. Wolfe R, Sharp L. Anti-vaccinationists past and present. BMJ. 2002;325(7361):430–2. https://doi.org/10.1136/bmj.325.7361.430.
28. Centers for Disease Control and Prevention. (2022). Smallpox/Monkeypox VIS. https://www.cdc.gov/vaccines/hcp/vis/vis-statements/smallpox-monkeypox.html
29. Duprex WP, Dutch RE. Paramyxoviruses: pathogenesis, vaccines, antivirals, and prototypes for pandemic preparedness. J Infect Dis. 2023;228(5):390–7. https://doi.org/10.1093/infdis/jiad123.
30. Haviid A, Rubin S, Muhlemann K. Mumps. Lancet. 2008;371:932–44. https://doi.org/10.1016/s0140-6736(08)60419-5.
31. U.S. Centers for Disease Control and Prevention. (2024). Clinical overview of mumps. https://www.cdc.gov/mumps/hcp/clinical-overview/?CDC_AAref_Val=https://www.cdc.gov/mumps/hcp.html
32. Yazigi A, De Pecoulas AE, Vauloup-Fellous C, Grangeot-Keros L, Ayoubi JM, Picone O. Fetal and neonatal abnormalities due to congenital rubella syndrome: a review of literature. J Matern Fetal Neonatal Med. 2017;30(3):274–8. https://doi.org/10.3109/14767058.2016.1169526.
33. McLean HQ, Fiebelkorn AP, Temte JL, Wallace GS, Centers for Disease Control and Prevention. Prevention of measles, rubella, congenital rubella syndrome, and mumps, 2013: summary recommendations of the Advisory Committee on Immunization Practices (ACIP). Morb Mortal Wkly Rep. 2013;62:1–34. https://www.cdc.gov/mmwr/preview/mmwrhtml/rr6204a1.htm

34. Strikas RA. Advisory committee on immunization practices recommended immunization schedules for persons aged 0 through 18 years—United States. Morb Mortal Wkly Rep. 2015;64(4):93–4. https://www.ncbi.nlm.nih.gov/pmc/articles/PMC4584857/
35. Wakefield A, Murch SH, Anthony A, Linnell J, Casson D, Malik M. Ileal-lymphoid-nodular hyperplasia, non-specific colitis, and pervasive developmental disorder in children (retracted). Lancet. 1998;351(9103):637–41. https://www.thelancet.com/journals/lancet/article/PIIS0140-6736(97)11096-0/fulltext
36. Godlee F, Smith J, Marcovitch H. Wakefield's article linking MMR vaccine and autism was fraudulent. BMJ. 2011;342 https://doi.org/10.1136/bmj.c7452.
37. Deer B. How the case against the MMR vaccine was fixed. BMJ. 2011;342 https://doi.org/10.1136/bmj.c5347.
38. Klein K, Diehl E. Relationship between MMR vaccine and autism. Ann Pharmacother. 2004;38(7–8):1297–300. https://doi.org/10.1345/aph.1d293.
39. Taylor B, Miller E, Lingam R, Andrews A, Simmons A, Stowe J. Measles, mumps, and rubella vaccination and bowel problems or developmental regression in children with autism: population study. BMJ. 2002;324(7334):393–5. https://doi.org/10.1136/bmj.324.7334.393.
40. Madsen K, Hviid A, Vestergaard M, Schendel D, Wohlfahrt J, Thorsen P, Olsen J, Melbey M. A population-based study of measles, mumps, and rubella vaccination and autism. N Engl J Med. 2002;347:1477–82. https://doi.org/10.1056/nejmoa021134.
41. Jain A, Marshall J, Buikema A. Autism occurrence by MMR vaccine status among US children with older siblings with and without autism. JAMA. 2015;313(15):1534–40. https://doi.org/10.1001/jama.2015.3077.
42. Public Health England. (2011). Completed primary courses at two years of age: England and Wales, 1966–1977, England only 1978 onwards. https://webarchive.nationalarchives.gov.uk/ukgwa/20140714111349/; http://www.hpa.org.uk/web/HPAweb&HPAwebStandard/HPAweb_C/1195733819251
43. McQuillen D, McQUillen M. Poliomyelitis. Elsevier Saunders; 2005.
44. Silverstein A, Silverstein A. Polio. Enslow Publishers; 2001.
45. World Health Organization. (2023). Poliomyelitis. https://www.who.int/news-room/fact-sheets/detail/poliomyelitis
46. Nathanson N, Langmuir AD. The cutter incident. Poliomyelitis following formaldehyde—inactivated poliovirus vaccination in the United States during the spring of 1955. Am J Trop Med Hyg. 1963;78:29–60. https://doi.org/10.1093/oxfordjournals.aje.a120328.
47. Offit P. The cutter incident, 50 years later. N Engl J Med. 2005;352:1411–2. https://doi.org/10.1056/nejmp048180.
48. Shah K, Nathanson N. Human exposure to SV40: review and comment. Am J Epidemiol. 1976;103(1):1–12. https://doi.org/10.1093/oxfordjournals.aje.a112197.
49. Thu G, Hem L, Hansen S, Moller B, Norstein J, Nokleby H, Grotmol T. Is there an association between SV40 contaminated polio vaccine and lymphoproliferative disorders? An age-period-cohort analysis on Norwegian data from 1953 to 1997. Int J Cancer. 2006;118(8):2035–8. https://doi.org/10.1002/ijc.21603.
50. Hmeljak J, Kern I, Cor A. No implication of simian virus 40 in pathogenesis of malignant pleural mesothelioma in Slovenia. Tumori. 2010;96(5):667–73. https://doi.org/10.1177/030089161009600504.
51. Qi F, Carbone M, Yang H, Gaudino G. Simian virus 40 transformation, malignant mesothelioma and brain tumors. Expert Rev Respir Med. 2011;5(5):683–97. https://doi.org/10.1586/ers.11.51.
52. Mohammad-Taheri Z, Nadji SA, Raisi F, Mohammadi F, Bahadori M, Mark E. No association between simian virus 40 and diffuse malignant mesothelioma of the pleura in Iranian patients: a molecular and epidemiologic case-control study of 60 patients. Am J Ind Med. 2013;56(10):1221–4. https://doi.org/10.1002/ajim.22160.
53. Petrovsky N, Aguilar JC. Vaccine adjuvants: current state and future trends. Immunol Cell Biol. 2004;82(5):488–96. Available. https://doi.org/10.1111/j.0818-9641.2004.01272.x.

54. Broder KR, Cortese MM, Iskander JK, Kretsinger K, Slade BA, Brown KH, Mijalski CM, Tiwari T, Weston EJ, Cohn AC, Srivastava PU, Moran JS, Schwartz B, Murphy TV, Advisory Committee on Immunization Practices (ACIP). Preventing tetanus, diphtheria, and pertussis among adolescents: use of tetanus toxoid, reduced diphtheria toxoid and acellular pertussis vaccines recommendations of the Advisory Committee on Immunization Practices (ACIP). Morb Mortal Wkly Rep. 2006;55:1–34. https://www.cdc.gov/mmwr/preview/mmwrhtml/rr5503a1.htm
55. National Institutes of Health. (n.d.) Tetanus. https://history.nih.gov/display/history/Tetanus
56. Acosta A, Moro P, Hariri S, Tiwari T. Chapter 7: Diptheria. 2024. https://www.cdc.gov/vaccines/pubs/pinkbook/dip.html
57. Ogden SA, Ludlow J, Alsayouri K. Diphtheria Tetanus Pertussis (DTaP) vaccine. StatPearls Publishing. https://www.ncbi.nlm.nih.gov/books/NBK545173/
58. Stephenson JB. A neurologist looks at neurological disease temporally related to DTP immunization. Tokai J Exp Clin Med. 1988;13(1):157–64. https://pubmed.ncbi.nlm.nih.gov/3078804/
59. Markowitz LE, Schiller JT. Human papillomavirus vaccines. J Infect Dis. 2021;224:367–78. https://doi.org/10.1093/infdis/jiaa621.
60. Jonson AL. Development of the human papillomavirus vaccine and guidelines for its use. J Ethics. 2007;9(1):30–3. https://doi.org/10.1001/virtualmentor.2007.9.1.cprl1-0701.
61. Bednarczyk RA. Addressing HPV vaccine myths: practical information for healthcare providers. Hum Vaccin Immunother. 2019;15(7–8):1628–38. https://doi.org/10.1080/21645515.2019.1565267.
62. Schlake T, Thess A, Fotin-Mleczek M, Kallen K. Developing mRNA-vaccine technologies. RNA Biol. 2012;9(11):1319–30. https://doi.org/10.4161/rna.22269.
63. Li M, Wang H, Tian L, Pang Z, Yang Q, Huang T, Fan J, Song L, Tong Y, Fan H. COVID-19 vaccine development: milestones, lessons and prospects. Signal Transduct Target Therapy. 2022;7(1):146. https://doi.org/10.1038/s41392-022-00996-y.
64. He Z, Su J, Ma Y, Zhang W, Tang S. A comprehensive analysis of the efficacy and effectiveness of COVID-19 vaccines. Front Immunol. 2022;13 https://doi.org/10.3389/fimmu.2022.945930.
65. Chung JY, Thone MN, Kwon YJ. COVID-19 vaccines: the status and perspectives in delivery points of view. Adv Drug Deliv Rev. 2021;170:1–25. https://doi.org/10.1016/j.addr.2020.12.011.
66. Mascellino MT, Di Timoteo F, De Angelis M, Oliva A. Overview of the main anti-SARS-CoV-2 vaccines: mechanism of action, efficacy, and safety. Infect Drug Resist. 2021;14:3459–76. https://doi.org/10.2147/IDR.S315727.
67. National Institutes of Health. (n.d.). Tetanus. https://history.nih.gov/display/history/Tetanus#:~:text=A%20method%20for%20inactivating%20tetanus,used%20during%20World%20War%20II
68. Canadian Institutes of Health Research. (2021). The long road to mRNA vaccines. https://cihr-irsc.gc.ca/e/52424.html
69. Liang Y, Huang L, Liu T. Development and delivery systems of mRNA vaccines. Front Bioengineering Biotechnol. 9 https://doi.org/10.3389/fbioe.2021.718753.
70. Rosner C, Genovese L, Tehrani B, Atkins M, Bakshi H, Chaudhri S, Damluji A, de Lamos J, Desai S, Emaminia A, Flanagan C, Khere A, Maghsoudi A, Mekonen G, Muthukumar A, Saeed I, Sherwood M, Sinha S, O'Connor C, deFillippi C. Myocarditis temporally associated with COVID-19 vaccination. Circulation. 2021;144(6) https://doi.org/10.1161/CIRCULATIONAHA.121.055891.
71. Centers for Disease Control and Prevention. (2022). Preventing and managing adverse reactions. https://www.cdc.gov/vaccines/hcp/acip-recs/general-recs/adverse-reactions.html
72. Food and Drug Administration. (2023). What is a serious adverse event?. https://www.fda.gov/safety/reporting-serious-problems-fda/what-serious-adverse-event
73. McNeil MM, DeStefano F. Vaccine-associated hypersensitivity. J Allergy Clin Immunol. 2018;141(2):463–72. https://doi.org/10.1016/j.jaci.2017.12.971.

74. Parker SK, Schwartz B, Todd J, Pickering LK. Thimerosal-containing vaccines and autistic spectrum disorder: a critical review of published original data. Pediatrics. 2004;114(3):793–804. https://doi.org/10.1016/B978-1-4557-0090-5.00076-8.
75. Offit PA, DeStefano F. Vaccine safety. Vaccine. 2013;2013:1464–80. https://doi.org/10.1016/B978-1-4557-0090-5.00076-8.
76. Goullé JP, Grangeot-Keros L. Aluminum and vaccines: current state of knowledge. Medecine et Maladies Infectieuses. 2020;50(1):16–21. https://doi.org/10.1016/j.medmal.2019.09.012.
77. Princip IN, Esposito S. Aluminum in vaccines: does it create a safety problem? Vaccine. 2018;36(39):5825–31. https://doi.org/10.1016/j.vaccine.2018.08.036.
78. Hassan SA, Wells RD, Davis CM. Egg hypersensitivity in review. Allergy & Asthma Proceedings. 2013;34(1):26–32.
79. Cox JE. Egg-based vaccines. Pediatric Rev. 2006;27(3):118–9. https://doi.org/10.1542/pir.27-3-118.
80. Gruenberg DA, Shaker MS. An update on influenza vaccination in patients with egg allergy. Curr Opin Pediatr. 2011;23(5):566–72. https://doi.org/10.2500/aap.2013.34.3621. https://doi.org/10.1097/mop.0b013e32834ac7a3
81. Tsai MH, Chiu CY. Allergic reactions to vaccines in children: from constituents to specific vaccines. Biomedicines. 2023;11(2):620. https://doi.org/10.3390/biomedicines11020620.

Chapter 2
Cultural Barriers

Archana Ramchandra Vatwani

2.1 Introduction

Protecting public health through increased vaccine uptake remains a priority in today's dynamic healthcare landscape, particularly in the context of global pandemics and the resurgence of infectious diseases. Vaccination, one of the most effective public health interventions, still faces challenges in achieving optimal uptake due to individual attitudes, social norms, and logistical barriers [9]. Disseminating accurate vaccine information and promoting immunization are crucial steps toward collective immunity and safeguarding vulnerable populations. However, cultural, socioeconomic, and operational challenges contribute to disparities in access and understanding, threatening global health goals.

Cultural barriers disproportionately impact marginalized communities, shaping attitudes toward vaccination. Social determinants of health and inequities play an essential role in the complex issues surrounding vaccination, influencing education and the acceptance of vaccines [7]. Geographical and cultural differences further complicate public health strategies, emphasizing the importance of tailored approaches to increase vaccine acceptance [28].

The scientific community has long acknowledged that many clinical trials fail to represent demographic diversity, leaving minorities underrepresented [11]. Patient safety concerns and public mistrust are significant implications of the lack of diversity in research studies. For example, an article from the Hopkins Biotech Network highlights the low number of African Americans recruited for COVID-19 treatment trials, despite being disproportionately affected by the pandemic [19]. Furthermore, not all research studies adequately account for the diverse needs of the population

A. R. Vatwani (✉)
Old Dominion University, Ellmer College of Health Sciences, Macon & Joan Brock Virginia Health Sciences at Old Dominion University, Norfolk, VA, USA
e-mail: avatwani@odu.edu

A. J. Chase et al. (eds.), *Vaccine Hesitancy Curriculum*,
https://doi.org/10.1007/978-3-031-88668-3_2

when considering treatments or interventions. Socioeconomic status, race, and ethnicity have been found to significantly influence COVID-19 infection and outcomes [20]. The COVID-19 Racial Data Tracker documented that the virus disproportionately impacted African Americans, Latinos, Hispanics, American Indians, and Native Americans [41].

The connection between people's beliefs, behaviors, and healthcare choices significantly impacts their attitudes toward health, their actions, and their perceptions of health-related matters. A wide variety of cultural factors—including differences in language, religious beliefs, and cultural norms—creates a complex backdrop that shapes and often restricts vaccination efforts. For this reason, healthcare providers must deeply understand cultural subtleties, as they are central to building trust in vaccines and ensuring equitable access for all individuals. By fostering trust and tailoring vaccine education to align with the cultural contexts and values of diverse populations, healthcare professionals can address and mitigate these disparities, increase vaccination rates, and promote health equity.

2.2 Research Questions

The pursuit of a comprehensive understanding of vaccine education and cultural barriers through a qualitative lens necessitates the formulation of three central questions:

- To what extent do cultural factors manifest as barriers to vaccine education and uptake among diverse populations?
- How do healthcare providers perceive and navigate cultural barriers to facilitate vaccine education and equitable access?
- What evidence-based strategies can effectively dismantle cultural barriers and enhance vaccine uptake within culturally diverse healthcare contexts?

These questions set up the framework for this chapter, aiming to pull out essential findings and empirical evidence.

2.3 Theoretical Frameworks

The Health Belief Model (HBM) is a theoretical and practical tool that can significantly enhance our understanding of individual health behavior decisions, including vaccination choices. This model suggests that a person's willingness to participate in health behavior, such as getting vaccinated, is influenced by how they view the risk and seriousness of the disease, the expected advantages of preventive actions, and the obstacles they may face. Key components also include cues to action, such as information from healthcare providers, and self-efficacy, which is the belief in one's ability to act [21, 30]. The HBM facilitates an analysis of how cultural beliefs influence perceptions related to vaccination, such as disease susceptibility and the benefits versus barriers of immunization. Utilizing the HBM, healthcare providers and policymakers can gain valuable insights into the factors influencing vaccination decisions, enabling them to develop strategies to address vaccine hesitancy effectively.

Another significant framework is the Theory of Planned Behavior (TPB), which broadens the understanding of individual actions by considering the impact of societal expectations and personal attitudes. The TPB suggests that an individual's actions are directly influenced by their intentions, which are shaped by attitudes toward the behavior, societal norms, and perceived control over the behavior [3]. This framework is precious for exploring how cultural norms and values mold attitudes toward vaccination and how perceived autonomy in the decision-making process influences vaccination decisions. By understanding the diverse influences on an individual's vaccination decision, healthcare providers and policymakers can develop comprehensive strategies that consider all these influences and promote vaccine uptake. Thus, by integrating cultural competence models, we can better understand the barriers to vaccine uptake and how to overcome them.

Literature evidence supports the effectiveness of various interventions in addressing vaccine hesitancy. A study on a culturally competent vaccine hesitancy educational model for community pharmacists demonstrated that a self-paced learning approach empowers pharmacists to develop effective strategies for increasing vaccine acceptance. Considering changing healthcare attitudes and behaviors, these interventions can reduce vaccine health disparities and enhance COVID-19 public health outcomes both locally and nationally [16]. Additionally, peer-based education interventions, where individuals from the same group act as vaccine educators, have shown potential in enhancing vaccination beliefs and increasing uptake, with effective strategies potentially involving a combined peer and healthcare expert approach [17].

These various approaches reinforce the essential need for developing culturally tailored public health strategies to enhance vaccine uptake on a global scale. Cultural competence models are essential frameworks that enable healthcare providers to effectively identify and address cultural barriers, fostering trust and improving communication with patients from diverse backgrounds. These models emphasize the importance of understanding the sociocultural dynamics that influence health behaviors, including vaccine hesitancy, and encourage healthcare providers to engage patients in a manner that is empathetic, respectful, and culturally appropriate. By employing culturally competent frameworks, healthcare providers can gain deeper insights into the complex interplay of individual beliefs, community norms, and systemic obstacles that contribute to vaccine hesitancy. This multifaceted approach recognizes that vaccine hesitancy is not solely a result of misinformation but is also shaped by historical, socioeconomic, and cultural factors. Furthermore, cultural competence models equip healthcare providers and policymakers with the tools needed to design educational interventions that go beyond simply delivering information. When integrated with public health policies, these models can help create inclusive vaccination programs that are accessible and equitable, ultimately reducing health disparities and improving overall public health outcomes. By embracing these principles, healthcare systems can address vaccine hesitancy more effectively, fostering higher vaccine acceptance rates and advancing global health equity.

2.4 Cultural Factors Influencing Vaccine Attitudes

Cultural factors can range from religious beliefs and mistrust of healthcare systems to traditional healing practices and language barriers. To develop successful vaccination campaigns and achieve high vaccination rates, it is essential to identify and address cultural factors, ensuring that healthcare interventions are culturally sensitive and tailored to the diverse populations they aim to reach. This approach not only fosters greater community engagement but also promotes better health outcomes on a global scale.

According to a narrative review by Wong et al., immigrants in Europe and North America encounter significant vaccine-related challenges, including misinformation and limited healthcare access. The study emphasizes the necessity of culturally sensitive healthcare and education tailored to these communities. It also calls for more research into the socioeconomic and cultural dynamics that contribute to vaccine hesitancy among immigrants to improve the effectiveness of vaccination programs [40].

The study "Applying Cultural Intelligence to Improve Vaccine Hesitancy Among Black, Indigenous, and People of Color" outlines the significance of healthcare providers considering the historical and cultural contexts that affect BIPOC communities' trust in medical advancements, including vaccines. It advocates for mindfulness and emotional intelligence to enhance patient–caregiver relationships, particularly when addressing vaccine hesitancy. These strategies and informed and respectful communication could enhance BIPOC individuals' openness to vaccination, potentially reduce COVID-19-related hospitalizations, and decrease fatalities [29].

An article by Shearn and Krockow discusses COVID-19 vaccine hesitancy and distrust toward medical interventions among ethnic and racial minority groups, including refugees, asylum seekers, and migrants. Themes include institutional mistrust, lack of confidence in the vaccine development process, and inadequate information from reliable sources, among other factors. The findings highlight the significant role of mistrust and call for culturally sensitive strategies to increase vaccine uptake [31].

Cultural influences, including historical events and the long-term development of vaccine-related attitudes, play a crucial role in shaping vaccine acceptability or resistance. Chile's successful vaccine rollout, despite limited resources and pandemic challenges, can be attributed to a well-established "vaccine culture." This acceptability is influenced by numerous factors, including historical events. This study by Ali [4] advocates for countries struggling with vaccination rates, suggesting that employing medical anthropologists could enhance public health strategies by integrating culturally relevant education, thus improving vaccine uptake and reducing the incidence of preventable diseases.

Similarly, a study by Dubé et al. [13] on strategies to address vaccine hesitancy indicates the complexity of the issue, emphasizing that no single intervention is universally effective. This highlights the need for multifaceted, data-driven, and culturally tailored approaches that address the unique concerns of diverse populations. The study also calls for rigorous evaluation and the sharing of insights to continuously refine strategies and enhance vaccine acceptance worldwide [13].

2.5 Access Disparities in Vaccine Uptake Among Underserved Populations

Cultural barriers and access disparities form a complex challenge in vaccine uptake, especially among underserved populations. These barriers are not only complex, involving social, logistical, and language-related issues, but are also profoundly intertwined, necessitating a comprehensive examination to devise effective mitigation strategies. Sociodemographic factors, such as income levels, play a significant role in the challenge of vaccine uptake. Lower income levels, for instance, are often associated with reduced healthcare access, including vaccinations. Financial constraints can limit transportation options to vaccination sites or the ability to take unpaid time off work. This economic barrier is further compounded in areas where healthcare resources are scarce, often in rural and some urban neighborhoods, resulting in fewer vaccination facilities and lower uptake rates [5, 6, 33, 34]. Furthermore, cultural attitudes and vaccine hesitancy play a significant role in shaping vaccine uptake, influencing both individual decisions and community-wide acceptance.

Historical and ongoing discrimination have fueled mistrust in the medical system among certain ethnic and racial groups, leading to skepticism about vaccine safety and efficacy. This issue is exacerbated by vaccine information and consent processes not being available in the patient's first language, which hampers understanding and trust [10]. A 2021 study by Tankwanchi et al. on vaccine hesitancy in migrant communities reveals that increased mobility and anti-immigrant sentiments exacerbate hesitancy, hindering efforts to prevent and eliminate communicable diseases [37]. Contributing factors include fears about vaccine safety, misinformation, language barriers and limited understanding of diseases and vaccines, distrust in local health systems, fear of deportation, limited physical access, and conflicts between vaccination and religious beliefs [1, 37].

A culturally sensitive, pharmacy-driven education program addressing COVID-19 vaccine hesitancy in individuals with mental illnesses successfully improved vaccination rates, particularly among underserved populations, with participants reporting an increased likelihood to vaccinate and high satisfaction with the program. This initiative highlights the effectiveness of tailored, pharmacist-led interventions in overcoming vaccine hesitancy barriers [23].

Moreover, despite generally adhering more to preventative practices, women show higher vaccine hesitancy, particularly regarding vaccine safety, which influences their decisions about vaccinations for their children [36]. Insurance coverage is another vital factor influencing vaccine access. The uninsured are less likely to receive vaccinations due to high out-of-pocket costs, and immigrants, especially those without legal status, often avoid vaccination due to fears of deportation or being ineligible for health insurance [22].

Vaccine-preventable diseases pose a substantial health risk, particularly to older adults, who are more vulnerable to functional decline, disability, or death from these infections. Factors influencing vaccination rates include sociodemographic aspects, logistical obstacles, cultural attitudes toward health literacy, and vaccine hesitancy. A comprehensive strategy is required, incorporating technology and communication, emphasizing physician-centered approaches, addressing systemic issues, and fostering political will and leadership [14].

Logistical barriers significantly contribute to vaccine hesitancy, particularly in areas with limited healthcare access and transportation. Limited healthcare access often results from an inadequate distribution of healthcare facilities, which can be incredibly sparse in rural or economically disadvantaged urban areas. More facilities are needed to make it easier for residents to obtain necessary vaccinations within a reasonable distance or timeframe. Transportation challenges further compound the issue of vaccine accessibility, particularly for individuals lacking personal vehicles or residing in areas with inadequate public transit systems. These logistical barriers not only impede access to vaccination sites but also deter individuals from seeking vaccinations due to the inconvenience, time commitment, and potential travel costs. To address these disparities, targeted interventions are needed to enhance healthcare accessibility, such as mobile vaccination units, subsidized transportation programs, and improvements in public transit infrastructure, ensuring equitable access to vaccines for underserved populations [5, 6, 33, 34].

2.6 Strategies for Dismantling Cultural Barriers to Vaccine Uptake

Enhancing vaccine access and uptake among ethnic minority and migrant communities requires building trust, reducing physical barriers, and improving communication about vaccine development. Trust can be fostered by acknowledging historical injustices and addressing concerns about exploitation in healthcare [1]. Transparency, accountability, and listening to community concerns are crucial [12]. A study looking at cultural competence as a strategy to address racial and ethnic health disparities in the United States recommends careful consideration of sociocultural barriers to care at organizational, structural, and clinical levels and proposes a framework of cultural competence interventions, including minority recruitment, interpreter services, culturally appropriate health materials, and cross-cultural provider education [8].

A literature review underscores diverse strategies to mitigate vaccine hesitancy, encompassing elements such as community health worker training, incentive-driven methods, advancements in health literacy facilitated by technology, and enhanced engagement with various media forms. These evidence-based approaches aim to increase vaccine acceptance and uptake through targeted and informed interventions. The following essential items are discussed:

2.6.1 Research and Policymaking

One significant barrier to research in general is the lack of diversity among research participants [38]. This issue is also pertinent in the development of state-level COVID-19 policies. Each study's methodology is unique and tailored to its inclusion and exclusion criteria, which are specific to the research objectives and may not represent the broader population. Research studies can only achieve full effectiveness by considering the diverse factors affecting treatment and interventions, as they must reflect the diversity of the public. Policymaking is an exceedingly complex process influenced by various political systems at different levels. Integrating research into health policy decisions enhances the process's effectiveness and efficiency by grounding it in evidence and scientific knowledge, thus benefiting both the research community and public health [25]. The use of research in formulating COVID-19 policies is facilitated by its foundation in evidence-based research and practice. Translating research studies into policies helps bridge the knowledge gap between the scientific community and the public, disseminating information in an accessible language that is comprehensible at various educational levels.

2.6.2 Culturally Tailored Outreach

Culturally tailored programs, often used synonymously with terms like culturally appropriate and cultural targeting, are interventions adapted to align with the cultural preferences and needs of specific populations, recommended to address and reduce health inequities [32]. Culturally tailored outreach is a vital strategy for overcoming vaccine hesitancy and dismantling barriers to immunization. This approach entails designing vaccine education and communication efforts specifically adapted to align with the cultural beliefs, values, and practices of diverse communities. Effective strategies include providing materials in multiple languages, incorporating cultural icons and narratives into communications, and respectfully addressing and dispelling common health beliefs and myths about vaccines across different cultures.

A study by Miguel et al. highlighted the impact of culturally tailored COVID-19 vaccine campaigns in local languages, including animated videos addressing misinformation distributed through social media platforms familiar to the community. This approach significantly increased COVID-19 vaccine uptake among indigenous populations in Guatemala [24]. Similarly, an initiative in West Virginia aimed at individuals living with chronic health conditions in rural areas addressed vaccine reluctance by offering educational tools and programs tailored to the community's cultural context. This strategy included brief informational videos produced by local healthcare professionals and interactive guides to facilitate discussions led by trained health navigators. These resources emphasized the importance of adapting health communication to the audience's cultural nuances and literacy levels [26].

A literature review identified significant barriers to vaccine acceptance in Latin America and the Caribbean region. These barriers included socioeconomic disadvantages, low education levels, lack of disease and vaccine awareness, and religious and cultural beliefs. The review emphasized that higher education levels and trust in healthcare professionals are crucial for improving vaccine uptake. To enhance vaccination coverage, the review suggested implementing educational programs for families and social mobilization strategies highlighting the benefits of vaccination and the risks associated with vaccine-preventable diseases. Additionally, it recommended providing adequate financial support and simplifying regulatory processes for introducing new vaccines [18]. Therefore, culturally tailored outreach increases vaccine uptake, fosters trust, and strengthens the relationship between healthcare providers and the communities they serve, ensuring that public health initiatives are more inclusive and effective.

2.6.3 Community Engagement and Collaborative Partnerships

Community engagement and involvement stand as pivotal pillars in dismantling cultural barriers to vaccine uptake, a process that has been robustly supported by extensive research demonstrating its effectiveness across diverse populations. Developing countries face challenges in reaching low-income and underserved communities for COVID-19 vaccination, exacerbated by mistrust due to the rapid development of vaccines. A study in Islamabad and Rawalpindi, Pakistan, using community engagement interventions, found that personalized information campaigns increased vaccine willingness by up to 7.6% in distant areas while improving access to vaccination services increased uptake by 17.1% in one treatment area, highlighting the need for localized and contextualized vaccination efforts [2].

An article describes a project partnered with faith-based organizations (FBOs) to promote COVID-19 vaccination, especially among vulnerable and marginalized communities. The project team worked with 18 FBOs and over 400 religious institutions to build confidence in the vaccination program, successfully facilitating the vaccination of 0.41 million beneficiaries [35]. Mobile clinics are essential in boosting vaccine uptake by bringing healthcare services directly to underserved communities, thus overcoming the access barrier of transportation. They offer essential medical care at lower costs, serving millions of at-risk individuals in the United States annually. Their adaptability during the COVID-19 pandemic, providing vaccines and other vital services, highlights their critical role in reducing healthcare disparities and enhancing public health [27].

Collectively, these studies demonstrate the importance of implementing community engagement strategies rooted in cultural competence, local leadership, and active participation in the design of health initiatives. A study focusing on increasing COVID-19 vaccine uptake employed a comprehensive strategy targeting Black and Hispanic youth, who face higher risks yet exhibit lower vaccination rates. This included engaging community partners, creating tailored handouts and posters, producing youth-centered videos, offering family-oriented vaccine information, training healthcare providers in effective communication, and using community health workers for counseling. The study developed effective intervention components by involving community partners to identify barriers and facilitators, significantly improving vaccine uptake through addressing specific community needs and promoting shared decision-making [15]. Such strategies are essential for effectively dismantling cultural barriers and enhancing vaccine uptake, ensuring that public health efforts are as inclusive as they are effective. Health campaigns can achieve broader reach and deeper impact through these multifaceted approaches, leading to higher vaccination rates and improved public health outcomes.

2.7 Discussion

The recurring themes identified in this chapter highlight the complexities surrounding vaccination decisions within culturally diverse settings. These findings illustrate the significant role of socioeconomic status in shaping vaccine hesitancy and refusal. Typically, individuals from marginalized communities, characterized by lower socioeconomic status, including reduced income and education levels, demonstrate pronounced vaccine hesitancy. In discussing the cultural barriers to vaccine uptake, it is crucial to consider how systemic inequities contribute to vaccine hesitancy across different socioeconomic groups. According to research highlighted in a 2023 publication, both privileged and marginalized communities exhibit vaccine hesitancy, though for different reasons rooted in systemic inequity. Marginalized groups often face barriers due to systemic disadvantages, such as limited healthcare access, which fosters mistrust and fear. Privileged groups, however, may perceive lower disease risk and exhibit a sense of autonomy over public health recommendations, which can also lead to vaccine hesitancy. This comprehensive perspective underscores the need for culturally sensitive strategies tailored to these diverse drivers of hesitancy to effectively enhance vaccine uptake [39]. This analysis highlights the necessity for approaches that address these determinants holistically, considering cultural context, income, and education as fundamental barriers to vaccine uptake. Furthermore, disparities in access to healthcare services across different cultures frequently emerge as a significant issue, necessitating a multifaceted approach to improving vaccine acceptance and coverage. Addressing these factors holistically is essential for mitigating the impacts of systemic inequity and enhancing public health outcomes.

Geographic, financial, and structural barriers impede access to vaccination services, leading to delayed or missed vaccinations. These barriers exacerbate health disparities, particularly among underserved populations. Linguistic diversity also poses a significant challenge, as individuals who face language barriers struggle to comprehend vaccination information and access healthcare resources. Therefore, culturally competent healthcare providers are essential in bridging these divides. Culturally tailored vaccine education and outreach strategies are crucial in addressing these issues.

Providing culturally sensitive messaging and interventions is pivotal in addressing vaccine hesitancy within diverse populations. Engaging community leaders and organizations that understand cultural nuances helps build trust and overcome barriers, including mistrust in healthcare systems rooted in historical injustices and discrimination. Cultural norms, values, beliefs, and practices significantly influence vaccine decision-making. In some cultural contexts, these factors may perpetuate vaccine hesitancy, while in others, they demonstrate resilience and resourcefulness in navigating barriers. Barriers like geographic, financial, and structural disparities disproportionately affect underserved populations, perpetuating health inequities.

Collaborative partnerships between healthcare providers and community organizations emerge as a central strategy. Engaging community-based organizations can bridge cultural divides and improve vaccine access. Policymakers should address access disparities, particularly in underserved communities, by investing in healthcare infrastructure, reducing financial barriers, and implementing policies that ensure equitable vaccine access. Recognizing geographic and structural factors contributing to disparities is essential. Healthcare providers should also prioritize health literacy initiatives and language services to bridge gaps in vaccine accessibility and education. Culturally competent healthcare providers play a pivotal role in building trust and addressing cultural barriers.

2.8 Conclusion

This chapter explored various cultural barriers to vaccine uptake within varied healthcare contexts. The synthesis of varied studies reveals consistent themes and challenges influencing vaccination decisions. The findings highlight the significant need for culturally tailored interventions. Socioeconomic disparities, language barriers, and cultural norms are significant in vaccine hesitancy. However, these barriers can be overcome through culturally sensitive education and outreach initiatives, including engaging with community partners, enhancing language services, and improving access to healthcare. More research studies on the social determinants of health examining the intersection of cultural barriers are required. Such investigations should also include monitoring changes in vaccine attitudes in response to new health policies and campaigns. By adopting a culturally competent approach and involving communities in the research process, we can advance toward equitable vaccine coverage and improved public health outcomes. Emphasizing cultural sensitivity in public health transcends being merely a moral imperative; it is a necessity for effective health intervention. Integrating cultural competence and cultural humility into public health efforts is essential for addressing the diverse needs of communities, thereby improving the accessibility and effectiveness of health services. This approach not only fosters understanding and respect for cultural differences but also encourages continuous growth among health professionals. By embracing respectful and informed practices, public health initiatives uphold ethical standards and achieve better health outcomes. These strategies empower individuals from all cultural backgrounds with the knowledge and support needed to make informed health decisions, ensuring that public health efforts are both practical and inclusive of the populations they serve.

References

1. Abba-Aji M, Stuckler D, Galea S, McKee M. Ethnic/racial minorities' and migrants' access to COVID-19 vaccines: a systematic review of barriers and facilitators. J Migr Health. 2022;5:100086. https://doi.org/10.1016/j.jmh.2022.100086.
2. Abdullah M, Ahmad T, Kazmi T, Sultan F, Afzal S, Safdar RM, Khan AA. Community engagement to increase vaccine uptake: quasi-experimental evidence from Islamabad and Rawalpindi, Pakistan. PloS One. 2022;17(12):e0274718. https://doi.org/10.1371/journal.pone.0274718.
3. Ajzen I. The theory of planned behavior. Organ Behav Hum Decis Process. 1991;50(2):179–211. https://doi.org/10.1016/0749-5978(91)90020-t.
4. Ali I. Culture of vaccine acceptability or resistance: the curious case of Chile's COVID-19 vaccine rollout and anthropology's role in increasing vaccination uptake. Vaccine. 2023;X, 13:100272. https://doi.org/10.1016/j.jvacx.2023.100272.
5. Anderson L. Economic barriers to vaccine access. J Public Health Policy. 2021a;42(1):13–25.
6. Anderson L. Addressing transportation barriers to healthcare access. J Health Dispar Res Pract. 2021b;14(2):112–29.
7. Bertoncello C, Ferro A, Fonzo M, Zanovello S, Napoletano G, Russo F, Baldo V, Cocchio S. Socioeconomic determinants in vaccine hesitancy and vaccine refusal in Italy. Vaccine. 2020;8(2):276. https://doi.org/10.3390/vaccines8020276.
8. Betancourt JR, Green AR, Carrillo JE, Ananeh-Firempong O. Defining cultural competence: a practical framework for addressing racial/ethnic disparities in health and health care. Public Health Rep. 2003;118(4):293–302. https://doi.org/10.1016/s0033-3549(04)50253-4.
9. Brewer NT, Chapman GB, Rothman AJ, Leask J, Kempe A. Increasing vaccination: putting psychological science into action. Psychol Sci Public Interest. 2017;18(3):149–207. https://doi.org/10.1177/1529100618760521. PMID: 29611455
10. Chen M, Lee P, Yang J. Cultural influences on vaccine acceptance. Cultural Health Insights. 2022;15(4):45–59.
11. Clark LT, Watkins L, Piña IL, Elmer M, Akinboboye O, Gorham M, Jamerson B, McCullough C, Pierre C, Polis AB, Puckrein G, Regnante JM. Increasing diversity in clinical trials: overcoming critical barriers. Curr Probl Cardiol. 2019;44(5):148–72. https://doi.org/10.1016/j.cpcardiol.2018.11.002.

12. Corbie-Smith G, Thomas SB, St. George DMM. Distrust, race, and research. Arch Intern Med. 2002, November 25;162(21):2458. https://doi.org/10.1001/archinte.162.21.2458.
13. Dubé E, Gagnon D, MacDonald NE. Strategies intended to address vaccine hesitancy: review of published reviews. Vaccine. 2015;33(34):4191–203. https://doi.org/10.1016/j.vaccine.2015.04.041.
14. Ecarnot F, Maggi S, Michel J. Strategies to improve vaccine uptake throughout adulthood. Vaccines for Older Adults: Current Practices and Future Opportunities; 2020. p. 234–48. https://doi.org/10.1159/000504486.
15. Enlow PT, Thomas C, Osorio AM, Lee M, Miller JM, Pelaez L, Kazak AE, Phan TLT. Community partnership to co-develop an intervention to promote equitable uptake of the COVID-19 vaccine among pediatric populations. Delaware J Public Health. 2024, March;10(1):30–8. https://doi.org/10.32481/djph.2024.03.06.
16. Gillard CJ, Al-Dahir S, Earls M, Singleton B. A culturally competent vaccine hesitancy educational model for community pharmacists to increase vaccine uptake, Louisiana, 2021–2022. Am J Public Health. 2022;112(S9):S900–3. https://doi.org/10.2105/ajph.2022.307070.
17. Gobbo ELS, Hanson C, Abunnaja KSS, et al. Do peer-based education interventions effectively improve vaccination acceptance? A systematic review. BMC Public Health. 2023;23:1354. https://doi.org/10.1186/s12889-023-16294-3.
18. Guzman-Holst A, DeAntonio R, Prado-Cohrs D, Juliao P. Barriers to vaccination in Latin America: a systematic literature review. Vaccine. 2020;38(3):470–81. https://doi.org/10.1016/j.vaccine.2019.10.088.
19. Haque W, Ahmadzada M. Lack of diversity in clinical trials: the problem and potential solutions. Hopkins Biotech Network; 2020, November 20. https://hopkinsbio.org/academic/diversity-in-clinical-trials/
20. Henry TA. Data from 10 cities show COVID-19 impact based on poverty, race. American Medical Association; 2020, August 5. https://www.ama-assn.org/delivering-care/health-equity/data-10-cities-show-covid-19-impact-based-poverty-race
21. Janz NK, Becker MH. The health belief model: a decade later. Health Educ Q. 1984;11(1):1–47. https://doi.org/10.1177/109019818401100101.
22. Johnson T. Insurance and legal barriers to vaccination. Vaccine Policy Rev. 2023;17(2): 110–24.
23. Liu I, Cruz A, Gamcsik S, Harris SC. Reducing barriers to COVID-19 vaccine uptake through a culturally sensitive pharmacy-led patient medication education group in a behavioral health population. J Am Pharm Assoc. 2023;63:915. https://doi.org/10.1016/j.japh.2023.01.012.
24. Miguel LA, Lopez E, Sanders K, Skinner NA, Johnston J, Vosburg KB, Diaz AK, Diamond-Smith N. Evaluating the impact of a linguistically and culturally tailored social media ad campaign on COVID-19 vaccine uptake among indigenous populations in Guatemala: a pre/post design intervention study. BMJ Open. 2022;12(12):e066365. https://doi.org/10.1136/bmjopen-2022-066365.
25. Mirvis DM. From research to public policy: an essential extension of the translation research agenda. Clin Transl Sci. 2009;2(5):379–81. https://doi.org/10.1111/j.1752-8062.2009.00144.x.
26. Misra R, Kirk B, Shawley-Brzoska S, Totzkay D, Morton C, Kuhn S, Harris M, McMillion M, Darling E. Educational intervention to increase COVID-19 vaccine uptake in rural patients with chronic diseases: lessons learned from an innovative academic–community partnership. Int J Environ Res Public Health/Int. 2024;21(1):71. https://doi.org/10.3390/ijerph21010071.
27. Mobile Clinics: A Powerful Resource for Addressing Health Disparities. (2020). https://info.primarycare.hms.harvard.edu/perspectives/articles/mobile-clinics-health-disparities

28. Reindl D, Catma S. A pre-vaccine analysis using the health belief model to explain parents' willingness to vaccinate (WTV) their children in the United States: implications for vaccination programs. Expert Rev Pharmacoecon Outcomes Res. 2022;22(5):753–61. https://doi.org/10.1080/14737167.2022.2045957.
29. Richard-Eaglin A, McFarland ML. Applying cultural intelligence to improve vaccine hesitancy among Black, indigenous, and people of color. Nurs Clin N Am. 2022;57(3):421–31. https://doi.org/10.1016/j.cnur.2022.04.008.
30. Rosenstock IM. Historical origins of the health belief model. Health Educ Monogr. 1974;2(4):328–35. https://doi.org/10.1177/109019817400200403.
31. Shearn C, Krockow EM. Reasons for COVID-19 vaccine hesitancy in ethnic minority groups: a systematic review and thematic synthesis of initial attitudes in qualitative research. SSM—Qualitative Research in Health. 2023;3:100210. https://doi.org/10.1016/j.ssmqr.2022.100210.
32. Singh H, Fulton J, Mirzazada S, Saragosa M, Uleryk EM, Nelson MLA. Community-based culturally tailored education programs for black communities with cardiovascular disease, diabetes, hypertension, and stroke: systematic review findings. J Racial Ethn Health. 2022;10(6):2986. https://doi.org/10.1007/s40615-022-01474-5.
33. Smith J, Gilbert S. Geographic disparities in healthcare resources and vaccination rates. Health Geogr. 2020a;38(3):222–31.
34. Smith J, Gilbert S. Healthcare accessibility and its impact on public health. Public Health Rev. 2020b;41(1):1–15.
35. Soni GK, Bhatnagar A, Gupta A, Kumari A, Arora S, Seth S, Rastogi A, Kanagat N, Fields R. Engaging faith-based organizations for promoting the uptake of COVID-19 vaccine in India: a case study of a multi-faith society. Vaccine. 2023;11(4):837. https://doi.org/10.3390/vaccines11040837.
36. Spees LP, Biddell CB, Angove RS, Gallagher KD, Anderson E, Christenbury A, Rocque G, Wheeler SB. Barriers to COVID-19 vaccine uptake among resource-limited adults diagnosed with chronic illness. Front Public Health. 2023;11 https://doi.org/10.3389/fpubh.2023.1046515.
37. Tankwanchi AS, Bowman B, Garrison M, Larson H, Wiysonge CS. Vaccine hesitancy in migrant communities: a rapid review of latest evidence. Curr Opin Immunol. 2021;71:62–8. https://doi.org/10.1016/j.coi.2021.05.009.
38. University of California San Francisco. (n.d.). Diversity in research participation: why it's important. https://recruit.ucsf.edu/diversity-research-participation-why-its-important
39. Vlasak D, Dinero RE, Roitman NA. Vaccine hesitancy at both ends of the socioeconomic spectrum: a new paradigm for understanding the role of systemic inequity. JPHE. 2023;10:10. https://doi.org/10.21037/jphe-23-81.
40. Wong J, Lao C, Dino G, Donyaei R, Lui R, Huynh J. Vaccine hesitancy among immigrants: a narrative review of challenges, opportunities, and lessons learned. Vaccine. 2024;12(5):445. https://doi.org/10.3390/vaccines12050445.
41. Wood D. (2020, September 23). As pandemic deaths add up, racial disparities persist—and in some cases worsen. NPR.org. https://www.npr.org/sections/health-shots/2020/09/23/914427907/as-pandemic-deaths-add-up-racial-disparities-persist-and-in-some-cases-worsen

Chapter 3
Medical Barriers to Vaccine Acceptance

Mayur S. Parmar and Cyril Blavo

3.1 Introduction

Vaccines have been developed to prevent more than 20 life-threatening diseases, helping people of all ages live longer, healthier lives. Immunization currently prevents 3.5–5 million deaths every year from diseases like diphtheria, tetanus, pertussis, influenza, COVID-19, and measles [1]. However, reluctance or refusal to vaccinate is threatening decades of progress in the global fight against infectious diseases.

Medical barriers to vaccine acceptance encompass a range of health-related concerns, misconceptions, and logistical challenges that hinder individuals from getting vaccinated. Significant focus is directed toward vaccine acceptance, particularly given that the World Health Organization (WHO) has classified vaccine hesitancy as a significant public health challenge [2]. These barriers are distinct from personal beliefs or philosophical objections and focus on medical information, safety concerns, and healthcare system factors. For instance, misinformation surrounding vaccines, such as measles, mumps, and rubella (MMR), and their link to autism, despite numerous studies disproving this claim, has significantly contributed to vaccine hesitancy [3]. Historically, overcoming medical barriers to vaccination has been successful, particularly through successfully eradicating diseases like poliomyelitis and smallpox.

Addressing medical barriers is crucial for improving vaccination rates and protecting the health of the public. When medical barriers are not adequately addressed, they can contribute to vaccine hesitancy, where individuals delay or refuse vaccines despite their availability. This hesitancy can lead to outbreaks of vaccine-preventable

M. S. Parmar (✉) · C. Blavo
Dr. Kiran C. Patel College of Osteopathic Medicine, Nova Southeastern University, Clearwater, FL, USA
e-mail: mparmar@nova.edu; cblavo@nova.edu

A. J. Chase et al. (eds.), *Vaccine Hesitancy Curriculum*,
https://doi.org/10.1007/978-3-031-88668-3_3

diseases, increased healthcare costs, and a higher burden on healthcare systems [2]. Such outbreaks can have devastating consequences, as evidenced by the 130% increase in global measles deaths between 2016 and 2019 [4]. Understanding barriers to vaccine acceptance in individuals is crucial to inform effective interventions for maximizing uptake. By identifying and mitigating these barriers, healthcare providers can build trust with patients, ensure equitable access to vaccines, and ultimately increase vaccination coverage, leading to better health outcomes. Community engagement is a crucial aspect of this process, connecting individuals and communities to achieve the overall goal of prevention [5–7].

This chapter delves into various aspects of medical barriers to vaccine acceptance, including the spread of medical misinformation and misunderstanding of vaccine safety and efficacy data. It explores how social media and unreliable sources contribute to misinformation, creating fear and distrust. The chapter also addresses concerns about vaccine ingredients and side effects, providing transparent explanations and differentiating between common side effects and rare adverse events. Additionally, it discusses true contraindications and necessary precautions, emphasizing individualized assessment by healthcare providers. Finally, the chapter examines access and delivery challenges, including geographic and financial barriers and healthcare system factors, highlighting the importance of clear communication, accurate information, and trust-building to overcome these barriers and improve vaccination rates.

3.2 Misinformation and Misunderstanding of Medical Information

3.2.1 The Spread of Medical Misinformation

In the digital age, social media has amplified medical misinformation and vaccine hesitancy through a variety of platforms and unreliable websites [8, 9]. False or misleading claims about vaccines, often lacking scientific basis, can rapidly disseminate and create fear, confusion, and distrust. This misinformation can range from misrepresentations about vaccine ingredients that exaggerated claims about side effects, ultimately deterring individuals from vaccination [9].

One prominent example is the misinformation surrounding the human papillomavirus (HPV) vaccine, which is an important vaccine that prevents HPV infections that may lead to cancers, such as anal, cervical, vaginal, vulvar, penile, and oropharyngeal [10, 11]. Antivaccine misinformation campaigns have disseminated false claims that the HPV vaccine causes infertility and primary ovarian insufficiency (POI) despite extensive research demonstrating its safety and efficacy in preventing several cancers [12]. Such misinformation creates fear and distrust, deterring individuals from vaccination and undermining public health efforts.

Similarly, misinformation about COVID-19 vaccines has been rampant. Claims that vaccines contain microchips for tracking or altering DNA have spread widely on social media [13]. Despite extensive scientific evidence confirming the safety and efficacy of COVID-19 vaccines, misinformation has fueled vaccine hesitancy. An example is the myth that mRNA vaccines can alter human DNA persists, even though mRNA does not integrate into the genome [13]. Other examples of misinformation about COVID-19 vaccines include claims that the vaccines were not tested appropriately prior to production. This misinformation has led to significant public fear and reluctance to receive the vaccine, hindering efforts to control the pandemic.

Addressing these forms of misinformation is crucial for improving vaccination rates and protecting the health of the public. Healthcare providers and public health officials must actively combat misinformation by providing accurate, evidence-based information and engaging with communities to build trust and dispel myths. By doing so, they can help ensure that individuals make informed decisions about vaccination based on reliable information rather than fear and falsehoods. CDC, WHO, American Academy of Pediatrics (AAP) and the Advisory Committee on Immunization Practices (ACIP) and WHO share information about various myths and facts about vaccinations to safeguard public health [13].

3.2.2 Misunderstanding of Vaccine Safety and Efficacy Data

Misconceptions about vaccine safety and efficacy are prevalent. Common misconceptions include the belief that vaccines cause autism despite overwhelming scientific evidence to the contrary. Addressing these misconceptions requires clear communication about the rigorous safety testing process that vaccines undergo before approval and transparent explanations of how vaccine efficacy is measured and interpreted.

A recent example involves the COVID-19 vaccines. Misinformation suggested that these vaccines were not evaluated in preclinical animal studies and were rushed directly into clinical trials. This misunderstanding was exacerbated by the rapid timeline of vaccine development, raising concerns about the thoroughness of the evaluation process. However, it is important to provide evidence that the mRNA technology used in COVID-19 vaccine development has been under evaluation for several years. The collaboration of multiple researchers worldwide and substantial government funding made the rapid development possible.

To gain public trust in vaccine safety and efficacy, it is crucial to highlight the comprehensive journey of vaccine development through literature writing and education [14]. This includes preclinical animal testing, all phases of clinical trials, and the rigorous regulatory review and approval process. Educating the public about these steps can help prevent misinformation and misunderstandings, ensuring that individuals make informed decisions based on accurate information.

3.3 Concerns About Vaccine Ingredients and Side Effects

3.3.1 Vaccine Ingredients

Transparency about vaccine ingredients is essential for addressing concerns, building trust, and overcoming vaccine hesitancy. Explaining the purpose of adjuvants, such as aluminum salts used in some vaccines to enhance immune response, can help dispel fears. Addressing specific concerns about thimerosal, a mercury-containing preservative removed from most childhood vaccines except for some influenza vaccines, is crucial for correcting misinformation. Vaccine ingredients can include adjuvants, preservatives, stabilizers, and residuals from the manufacturing process. Adjuvants such as aluminum salts are used to enhance the immune response. Preservatives like thimerosal are used to prevent bacterial growth, and stabilizers like sugars are used to maintain the vaccine's potency. Each component is specific in ensuring the vaccine's safety and efficacy.

The Center for Biologics Evaluation and Research (CBER) of the U.S. Food and Drug Administration (FDA) plays a crucial role in the approval and quality control of vaccine ingredients [15, 16]. CBER ensures that biological products, including vaccines, are safe, effective, and of high quality. This includes overseeing the vaccine development process, from preclinical studies to clinical trials, and ensuring that all vaccine ingredients meet stringent safety and efficacy standards. This rigorous regulatory process provides reassurance to the public and healthcare professionals.

Adjuvants are substances added to vaccines to enhance the body's immune response to the antigen and are categorized as immunostimulants and delivery systems. These adjuvants can help administer lesser quantities of the vaccine and fewer doses [17]. Some common adjuvants used are aluminum salts, monophosphoryl A, saponin (QS21), CpG, and squalene [17]. One common adjuvant is aluminum salts, which have been used in several vaccines, such as hepatitis A, hepatitis B, and pneumococcal vaccines. Adjuvants are not used in live viral vaccines, such as rubella, varicella, measles, mumps, and rotavirus [18]. Aluminum salts help create stronger and longer-lasting immunity by stimulating the immune system to respond more vigorously to the vaccine. Before an adjuvant is selected as a vaccine ingredient, extensive research is done for its safety and side effects.

Preservatives prevent microbial growth and contamination and ensure the vaccine remains safe and effective over time [19]. Thimerosal, a mercury-containing preservative, was once commonly used in vaccines. However, due to public concerns, thimerosal has been removed from most childhood vaccines since the early 2000s, except for some multi-dose FDA-approved seasonal influenza vaccines [19]. Due to the concern and fear among parents that thimerosal contained in vaccines might harm their children, numerous studies have been conducted (larger and controlled studies) demonstrating that thimerosal in the amounts used in vaccines is not harmful [19]. Today, many vaccines (U.S. FDA-licensed vaccines) are packaged, reformulated, and developed in single-use presentations, resulting in a decline in thimerosal use as a preservative, hence minimizing the number of preservative ingredients added to the vaccine.

Stabilizers such as sugars, gelatin, and proteins are added to vaccines to protect them from adverse conditions like heat, light, and acidity, ensuring they remain effective during storage and transportation. These stabilizers are carefully selected and tested for safety.

Residuals from the manufacturing process, such as trace amounts of antibiotics or egg proteins, may be present in some vaccines. These residuals are present in extremely low quantities and are not harmful. For example, some vaccines are produced using chicken eggs, which can leave trace amounts of egg protein in the final product. Although most people with egg allergies can safely receive these vaccines, this is important for individuals with severe egg allergies to consider.

By addressing specific concerns about vaccine ingredients and providing clear and accurate educational information about their purpose and safety, healthcare providers can help dispel fears and encourage vaccination. As vaccine ingredients are an important barrier to vaccine hesitancy, accurate and easily accessible information is crucial for correcting misinformation and building public trust.

3.3.2 Side Effects and Adverse Events

Differentiating between common, mild side effects and rare, serious adverse events is important for contextualizing vaccine safety. Common side effects, such as soreness or low-grade fever, are typically temporary and indicate a normal immune response. Serious adverse events are rare and monitored through robust reporting systems like the Vaccine Adverse Event Reporting System [20]. Discussing the risks and benefits of vaccination by healthcare professionals allows individuals to make informed decisions based on accurate information.

3.4 Contraindications and Precautions

3.4.1 Contraindications

Contraindications to vaccination are rare and specific medical conditions that make vaccination unsafe for an individual. These may include severe allergic reactions to previous doses or to specific vaccine components. The healthcare provider's role is crucial in determining contraindications based on individual medical histories and ensuring that vaccines are administered safely. Hence, taking the most accurate or detailed individual medical histories is crucial during vaccination.

3.4.2 Precautions

Precautions are situations where vaccination may be recommended cautiously or after careful consideration. Pregnant individuals may be advised to receive certain vaccines, such as the Tdap vaccine, at specific times during pregnancy to maximize protection for both mother and baby. Healthcare providers must consider individual circumstances to determine the best course of action, weighing vaccination's potential risks and benefits on a case-by-case basis.

3.5 Access and Delivery Challenges

3.5.1 Geographic and Financial Barriers

Individuals in rural or underserved areas may face geographic barriers to accessing vaccines, such as long distances to healthcare facilities or limited availability of providers. Financial barriers, such as high out-of-pocket costs for uninsured individuals, can deter vaccination. Addressing these barriers requires expanding access through mobile clinics, community outreach programs, and establishing policies like the Vaccines for Children (VFC) program, which provides free vaccines to eligible children ages 18 years and younger [21].

The goal of the VFC in the United States is to provide vaccines to children whose parents or guardians may not be able to afford them. The goal is to improve vaccine access nationwide at no cost to VFC-program-eligible children through VFC-program-enrolled public and private healthcare providers. Under this program, children who are 18 years old or younger who meet at least one of the following criteria are eligible: American Indian or Alaska Native, Medicaid-eligible, uninsured, or underinsured [21]. Public health educational programs and healthcare personnel can play an important role in making this information available to eligible guardians. Such programs have been crucial in overcoming financial barriers and protecting children from several diseases and have saved nearly $2.2 trillion in preventing illness [21].

3.5.2 Healthcare System Factors

Healthcare system factors, like vaccine shortages or inadequate provider training, can impede vaccination efforts. During the COVID-19 pandemic, ensuring equitable distribution and adequate supply of vaccines was a significant challenge. Educating healthcare providers about the latest vaccine recommendations and streamlining vaccination delivery processes are essential for overcoming these barriers.

3.6 Addressing Medical Barriers

Overcoming medical barriers requires a multifaceted approach:

- *Clear communication:* Healthcare providers must communicate clearly and empathetically, address concerns, correct misinformation, and provide accurate vaccine information.
- *Trust-building:* Building trust between healthcare providers and patients is crucial. Open dialogue, transparency, and respectful interactions can foster trust and encourage vaccine acceptance.
- *Public health campaigns:* Educational campaigns that provide accurate information, address misconceptions, and promote the benefits of vaccination can reach a broad audience and encourage informed decision-making. Such public health awareness research-based messages can be delivered utilizing advertisement boards, TV, radio, print, and currently available social media platforms. These media should be culturally and linguistically competent.

A national program of the U.S. Department of Health and Human Services (HHS), the Pan Respiratory Virus (PRV) Public Education Campaign (PEC), also called "Risk Less. Do More," has been increasing awareness of and confidence in vaccine uptake that can potentially reduce the incidence of severe illnesses, such as influenza, COVID-19, and the Respiratory Syncytial Virus (RSV) in at-risk populations [5]. During the recent COVID-19 pandemic, a successful public education campaign, "We Can DO This," was crucial in not only saving individual lives but also an estimated net benefit of $731.9 billion in societal benefits due to averted illness and related costs [6, 22].

Overall, public health information campaigns help to educate the population about effective prevention measures against severe illnesses mediated by microorganisms that can be prevented through vaccination, overcome misinformation and misunderstanding, and enhance trust in vaccines.

- *Community engagement:* Engaging with communities, addressing their concerns, and partnering with trusted community leaders can increase vaccine confidence and acceptance.
  The Administration for Community Living (ACL) program has played a significant role in encouraging vaccination among older individuals, particularly during the COVID-19 pandemic [7]. Grants are awarded to organizations nationwide to support vaccination efforts, especially for older adults and people with disabilities. Activities funded include community outreach, educational campaigns, running vaccine clinics and mobile vaccination units, transportation assistance to vacation sites, and in-home vaccination services. The CDC-funded REACH Program (Racial and Ethnic Approaches to Community Health) has been instrumental in working with communities to reduce health disparities. Between 2001 and 2009, the REACH program reported increased vaccination rates among various population groups. Pneumonia vaccination rates rose from 50.5% to 60.5% in Black communities, from 46.0% to 58.5% in Hispanic communities, from 37.5% to 59.7% in Alaska Native and Pacific Islander communities, and from 67.3% to 78.7% in American Indian communities [23].

3.7 Conclusion

Medical barriers to vaccine acceptance pose significant challenges to public health prevention efforts. By addressing misinformation, clarifying concerns about safety and efficacy, and improving access to vaccines, we can overcome these barriers and increase vaccination rates. Continued research, open communication, and collaboration between healthcare providers, public health officials, and communities are essential for building a future where vaccines are widely accepted and appropriately utilized to protect individuals and communities from preventable diseases.

References

1. Vaccines and immunization. World Health Organization. Vaccines and Immunization. Accessed 10 Dec 2024
2. Kaufman J, Tuckerman J, Bonner C, et al. Parent-level barriers to uptake of childhood vaccination: a global overview of systematic reviews. BMJ Glob Health. 2021;6(9) https://doi.org/10.1136/bmjgh-2021-006860.
3. Bezbaruah R, Sailo N, Zonunmawii DK, Bhutia YD, Kakoti BB. Myths and facts about vaccination: dispelling myths and misconceptions with science. In: Advanced vaccination technologies for infectious and chronic diseases. Academic Press; 2024.
4. Durrheim DN, Andrus JK, Tabassum S, Bashour H, Githanga D, Pfaff G. A dangerous measles future looms beyond the COVID-19 pandemic. Nat Med. 2021;27(3):360–1. https://doi.org/10.1038/s41591-021-01237-5.
5. Risk Less. Do More. U.S. Department of Health and Human Services (HHS). Accessed 10 Dec 2024. https://www.hhs.gov/risk-less-do-more
6. We Can Do This. Accessed 10 Dec 2024. https://www.hhs.gov/risk-less-do-more
7. Administration for Community Living. Vaccination Resources. Administration for Community Living. Updated 08/13/2024. Vaccination Resources ACL Administration for Community Living. Accessed 10 Dec 2024
8. Puri N, Coomes EA, Haghbayan H, Gunaratne K. Social media and vaccine hesitancy: new updates for the era of COVID-19 and globalized infectious diseases. Hum Vaccin Immunother. 2020;16(11):2586–93. https://doi.org/10.1080/21645515.2020.1780846.
9. Ayaz H, Celik MH, Koytak HZ, Yanik IE. Exploring vaccine hesitancy in digital public discourse: from tribal polarization to socio-economic disparities. PLoS One. 2024;19(11):e0308122. https://doi.org/10.1371/journal.pone.0308122.
10. Liebermann E, Kornides M, Matsunaga M, et al. Use of social media and its influence on HPV vaccine hesitancy: US National Online Survey of mothers of adolescents, 2023. Vaccine. 2024:126571. https://doi.org/10.1016/j.vaccine.2024.126571.
11. Massey PM, Kearney MD, Hauer MK, Selvan P, Koku E, Leader AE. Dimensions of misinformation about the HPV vaccine on Instagram: content and network analysis of social media characteristics. J Med Internet Res. 2020;22(12):e21451. https://doi.org/10.2196/21451.
12. Smith TC, Gorski DH. Infertility: a common target of antivaccine misinformation campaigns. Vaccine. 2024;42(4):924–9. https://doi.org/10.1016/j.vaccine.2024.01.043.
13. Myths and Facts about COVID-19 Vaccines. Centers for Disease Control and Prevention Updated 02/16/2023. Myths and Facts about COVID-19 Vaccines CDC Archive.
14. Khehra N, Padda I, Jaferi U, Atwal H, Narain S, Parmar MS. Tozinameran (BNT162b2) vaccine: the journey from preclinical research to clinical trials and authorization. AAPS PharmSciTech. 2021;22(5):172.

15. Vaccine. Food and Drug Administration. Updated 01/12/2024. Vaccines FDA.
16. Center for Biologics Evaluation and Research (CBER). Food and Drug Administration. Updated 09/18/2024. Center for Biologics Evaluation and Research (CBER) FDA.
17. Zhao T, Cai Y, Jiang Y, et al. Vaccine adjuvants: mechanisms and platforms. Signal Transduct Target Ther. 2023;8(1):283. https://doi.org/10.1038/s41392-023-01557-7.
18. Vaccine Ingredients. Children's Hospital of Philadelphia. Updated December 15, 2022. https://www.chop.edu/vaccine-education-center
19. Thimerosal and Vaccines. Updated 02/01/2018. Thimerosal and Vaccines FDA. Accessed 10 Dec 2024
20. Vaccine Adverse Event Reporting System (VAERS). U.S. Department of Health and Human Services (HHS). Vaccine Adverse Event Reporting System (VAERS). Accessed 10 Dec 2024
21. About the Vaccines for Children (VFC) Program. Centers for Disease Control and Prevention. https://www.cdc.gov/vaccines-for-children
22. Turner S, Kranzler EC, Trigger S, et al. Benefit-cost analysis of the HHS COVID-19 Campaign: April 2021–March 2022. Am J Prev Med. 2024;67(2):258–64. https://doi.org/10.1016/j.amepre.2024.03.018.
23. REACH Program impact | REACH | CDC. Ctr Dis Control Prev. https://www.cdc.gov/reach. Accessed 10 Dec 2024

Chapter 4
Active Learning to Improve Vaccine Uptake: Educate, Motivate, and Vaccinate

Aarti Raja and Bharat S. Krishna

In public health, vaccination is considered one of the most effective and cost-efficient interventions. According to the World Health Organization (WHO), vaccination can prevent two to three million deaths annually worldwide (WHO 2019). Yet, in many regions of the world, vaccination is rejected, questioned, or inaccessible to the population. These issues already existed before 2020. However, the arrival of the COVID-19 pandemic and widespread access to information via the internet and social media brought new challenges concerning vaccine uptake to light. There have been many advances related to vaccine program development; however, an immunization program can only be successful if vaccine uptake is effective. As a result, in an era of vaccine skepticism and pandemic threats, there is a need to develop interventions that will promote vaccine uptake and reduce apprehension toward vaccinations. Of course, the foundation for any vaccine uptake and program should include high-quality clinical evidence but the focus of vaccine promotion programs could shift from data to other strategies that will impact people's behavior. This chapter centers on how health professionals can address vaccine hesitancy using active learning approaches.

A. Raja (✉)
Department of Biological Sciences, Halmos College of Arts and Sciences,
Nova Southeastern University, Fort Lauderdale, FL, USA
e-mail: araja@nova.edu

B. S. Krishna
C.I.T.I. Program, New York, NY, USA
e-mail: BKrishna@citiprogram.org

A. J. Chase et al. (eds.), *Vaccine Hesitancy Curriculum*,
https://doi.org/10.1007/978-3-031-88668-3_4

4.1 A Brief History and Context for Vaccine Hesitancy

In 2019, the WHO listed vaccine hesitancy as one of the leading threats to global health (WHO 2019). The WHO's experts note that the vaccine hesitancy issue is complex and context-specific, varying across time, place, and types of vaccines. It is influenced by misinformation, complacency, convenience, and confidence. Based on the definition of vaccine hesitancy, it is evident that hesitancy is a spectrum ranging from complete rejection of vaccine use to delaying its use. There are many models based on behavioral science, bioethics, and economics that can help us understand the factors contributing to vaccine hesitancy. Several factors, such as misinformation, mistrust, social norms, and personal beliefs, can influence vaccine hesitancy [1, 2]. We must recognize heterogeneity in vaccine-hesitant individuals and the various situations surrounding their hesitancy. Therefore, there is likely no "one-size-fits-all" approach, and interventions to address vaccine hesitancy must be context-specific and problem-specific [1, 2].

Data from a survey conducted across 24 countries (a mix of countries from Asia and the West) to understand the underlying roots of vaccine hesitancy and attitudes showed value-based differences in political thought that lead to differences in policies and beliefs in a population [50]. The study shed light on the idea that interventions must go beyond focusing on individual-level access to information and simply correcting myths about vaccinations in general. Public health researchers identified four main values associated with vaccine hesitancy: conspiratorial thinking, reactance, disgust sensitivity (toward needles or the idea of getting an illness), and individual worldviews. The consistency of these value associations across diverse geographies and populations informs us about the type of strategies we must develop to improve vaccine uptake. If intervention strategies can address the above values, the possibility of advancing vaccine confidence may be improved.

The best way to battle misinformation is to replace it with trustworthy, solid, science-based, understandable information communicated clearly, honestly, and consistently from a trustworthy source. This is the primary priority recently articulated by incoming CDC Director Dr. Mandy Cohen [3]. Given the abundance of available information, it becomes essential to understand the sources people use and get their scientific information. It has been shown that people most likely get their health information from primary care providers, nurses, family, medical websites, online search engines, specialist doctors, and friends, in that order. Previous studies also reported that health professionals and the Internet were the most frequently used sources for health information, and primary care providers were the most trusted sources [4, 5]. With the rise in the use of online information and the risk of spreading misinformation worldwide combined with the recent increase in vaccine-preventable diseases, it is imperative to ensure health professionals develop the appropriate skills and are equipped to communicate well-supported medical science concepts effectively. The responsibility tends to fall to the medical community to build people's trust in science and the scientific process. In an era with abundant information, it becomes necessary to distill content with scientific merit and present it to the people in need in a culturally sensitive manner.

An extensive review of intervention tools used by healthcare providers to educate patients in North America demonstrated that interventions mainly focus on knowledge sharing and communication training. The review identified areas that can be improved, and the unmet needs of the intervention tools were listed as:

- Ensuring the intervention is accessible
- The intervention must address multiple disciplines of medical specialties that are involved in vaccine discussions
- A method must exist to monitor physicians' and other health professionals' efforts and evaluate how clinicians manage difficult conversations surrounding vaccines

Beyond providing information, access to vaccines must be improved. This is especially true in middle-low-income countries. Even in developed nations, there might be areas that are underserved with regard to healthcare access. Ensuring strategies are in place to provide equitable access to vaccines to all people remains a global challenge. This can include campaigns such as mobile health clinics, training health care personnel in vaccine-related information delivery, vaccine delivery, development of cost-effective vaccines, and establishing programs that address social determinants of health barriers to promote equitable access. This would require the concerted efforts of those delivering the vaccines and investment in vaccine development from governmental and pharmaceutical/biotechnology companies. This is a challenging task with many competing interests. Still, it must include elements of vaccine security (the UNICEF and WHO define vaccine security as the timely, sustained, uninterrupted supply of affordable, assured quality vaccines), potentially in the form of regional manufacturing that produces an affordable, predictable supply of quality vaccines that reflect the needs of the local community while balancing the challenges of demand for vaccination [6]. Engagement of countries and agencies within a country (state and nonstate) in a defined shared vision will help implement such programs.

4.2 What Interventions Have (Not) Worked in the Past to Address Vaccine Hesitancy?

Programs developed around vaccination often include subject matter related to vaccine safety, the study of vaccines, and, at times, interpersonal communication skills. While vaccine administration training is included in the curriculum of several health professionals, it is not universally incorporated into the medical school preclinical curriculum [56]. Health professionals must be trained and updated on the effective methodologies for vaccination programs from an early stage in their careers.

Designing training programs that include patient education, building community confidence, administering vaccines, and educating trainees on the commonly encountered myths/misperceptions (and how to counter them) from the early stages of training could help address issues with vaccine hesitancy. These programs can begin in medical or nursing school or pharmacy school and continue throughout the practice tenure of the health professionals. Physicians and health professionals can currently take many courses as part of continuing medical education (CME) or continuing education (CE) programs to increase their knowledge and skills and stay up to date with the changing landscape of medicine. Introducing CME and CE focused on vaccine hesitancy and helping improve trust in science can serve as one avenue by which health professionals can advance their understanding of this issue and thereby aid in vaccine uptake. Courses such as "Understanding Vaccine Acceptance & Strategies to Increase Vaccine Uptake from the European Centre for Disease Prevention and Control," "Communicating Research Findings from CITI Program," and You Call the Shots by the Centers for Disease Control" are examples of e-learning options available for the healthcare provider community [51–53].

In 2017, a report was developed by the London School of Hygiene and Tropical Medicine Vaccine Confidence Project as part of the European Center for Disease Prevention and Control (ECDC) initiative to provide tools to address vaccine hesitancy [7]. The authors highlighted various practical tools for public health organizations and immunization stakeholders to address the challenging problem of vaccine hesitancy. The report outlined 40 interventions; the majority (27 of 40) used communication, dialogue, or tools for parents and healthcare professionals to aid health literacy. Ten of the interventions were diagnostic tools for monitoring and surveillance. The remaining interventions were advocacy campaigns and reminder–recall systems designed to remind patients and healthcare professionals about vaccination—the interventions aimed to combat misinformation and safety concerns and to overcome vaccine hesitancy.

The WHO's Strategic Advisory Group of Experts on Immunization (SAGE) working group published two reviews: January 2007–October 2013 [8] and January 2008–November 2014 [9]. These reviews highlighted that interventions employing multiple strategies were the most effective. Strategies were (1) directly targeting unvaccinated or under-vaccinated populations [10]; (2) increasing vaccination knowledge and awareness [11]; (3) improving convenience and access to vaccination [12]; (4) targeting specific populations (e.g., healthcare professionals) [13]; (5) mandating vaccinations or sanctions against nonvaccination [14]; and (6) engaging religious or other influential leaders to promote vaccination [15]. Targeting interventions to specific populations and their concerns was the most effective. Interventions that focused on quality improvement at clinics (e.g., improved data collection and monitoring, extended clinic hours, passive interventions (e.g., posters, websites), and incentive-based interventions using conditional or unconditional cash transfers were not as successful (had less than 10% increase in vaccine uptake) [8]. Interventions that showed a positive impact involved social mobilization, mass media and communication-based training for healthcare professionals, and nonfinancial incentives [8].

A caveat remains that the above studies (SAGE and ECDC) were conducted in high-income countries and cannot serve as generalized recommendations. Interventions must be developed and assessed within low-to-middle-income countries as well. The WHO has designed the behavioral and social drivers (BeSD) tools and survey instruments that many countries can use to evaluate reasons for poor vaccine uptake in childhood for COVID-19 [55]. This can serve as a blueprint for other vaccine campaigns to counter misconceptions around vaccines and vaccine-preventable diseases.

Health professionals at all stages of their careers will benefit from approaches to addressing vaccine-related communication early in their education. Recently, the Surgeon General's report called on educators to focus on strengthening and scaling up evidence-based programs that will build resilience to misinformation [16]. Interventions should be tailored to specific groups rather than the population at large. To accomplish this, measurement of vaccine hesitancy is key. Several tools have been developed to measure parent/caregiver hesitancy about childhood vaccination [54], but validated tools do not exist to measure adult vaccine hesitancy. The WHO is developing standardized quantitative and qualitative tools to measure drivers of vaccination [17]. It is vital to learn along the way to combat vaccine hesitancy and bring about changes. Policy actions must inform our learning so that policies are tested and refined in real time. Still, knowing that education is valuable, we should also take actions that speed up learning. In other words, "learn as you act and act to learn." This involves incorporating active learning strategies to help increase vaccine adoption.

4.3 What Type of Active Learning Session May Help with Future Interventions?

Several active learning strategies have been utilized to combat misinformation and vaccine hesitancy [16, 18]. Building upon these multi-pronged approaches and utilizing similar strategies are imperative to increase vaccine acceptance. Many studies have shown that actively engaging all the stakeholders in a population is crucial to achieving good vaccine acceptance. The parties involved must be appropriately trained to understand the population they will be serving. It has been shown that physicians are the most trusted messengers in delivering vaccine information. But depending on the location, multiple people could act as messengers delivering information about vaccines and their effectiveness and/or in administering vaccines. Health professionals must be trained to deliver consistent messaging to the patients we serve based on recommendations from locally active health agencies that are pertinent to the local population.

Strategies, therefore, must include the following:

4.3.1 Communication

Broad vaccination campaigns can generally influence a community's attitudes toward vaccination. However, since vaccine hesitancy sits on a spectrum, designing tailored communications to reach vulnerable populations will be better served. To achieve this, vaccine communication must be context-specific and evidence-based and take cultural issues into account. This will ensure discussions are focused and, therefore, more likely to be productive. Vaccine communication from health professionals will be crucial to achieving success. This communication/discussion should center on fostering receptivity and not reactivity. These professionals must be equipped with tools and training to engage effectively with people and generate receptivity.

A good example is a plan designed by the government of Canada [19]. The Council of Canadian Academies Expert Panel on Health Product Risk Communication Evaluation recognized that many of the existing communication products used by health professionals could be improved to better align with evidence-based communication best practices. The committee identified five best practices:

1. First, identify the target audience and establish trust.
2. Second, provide both the risks and benefits of vaccination, as most people seek balanced information.
3. Third, give the facts before addressing the myths.
4. Fourth, use visual aids.
5. Fifth, test communication material before launch.

Their recommendation was to apply these best practices to current or future communication products to aid vaccine providers (including physicians, nurse practitioners, pharmacists, and public health professionals) in developing communication materials that are sensitive to the complex ways that people process information and thus more likely to optimize vaccine uptake in their communities. All these suggestions were provided via materials such as websites, factsheets, posters, videos, etc. These were updated regularly and published on the government website CanVax.

When health professionals have conversations, motivational interviewing provides a more structured approach to guide people toward change by enhancing their internal rationale. This educational intervention takes 15–20 min and uses simple, understandable language to encourage discussion and questions from patients rather than provide prescriptive information. This has been demonstrated in regional studies in the UK, where there was a 12% increase in parents' intention to vaccinate and a 40% decrease in vaccination hesitancy scores following the intervention [20]. Another study in the United States around HPV vaccine communication, which included motivational interviewing, concluded that there was improved HPV vaccine series initiation and completion (a 9.5-absolute percentage point increase in HPV vaccine series initiation and a 4.4-absolute percentage point increase in HPV vaccine series completion in intervention practices) among adolescent patients [21].

Another method advocated combines a presumptive approach to conversations with teachable methods to foster receptivity and trust in conversations [22]. The main idea showcases that it is necessary to put human relationships at the center of vaccine acceptance conversations to build trust in vaccination. Termed AIMS, the method for vaccination conversations involved the following four steps:

- Announce: announce that vaccination will happen, assuming people are ready for it.
- Inquire: use open-ended discussions to review patient concerns.
- Mirror: reflect back to make the person feel heard.
- Secure: consolidate the conversation by securing trust.

Health professionals' communication methods could include the teach-back method and plain language when interacting with patients with lower health literacy [23]. Health professionals could apply strategies such as creating easy-to-understand brief messages that can be delivered via television and include newer avenues such as online platforms, blogs, and websites. They could employ celebrity branding to increase the use of and trust in credible medical websites and government sources.

These communication methodologies can be used by any health professional delivering vaccine information and are not limited to physicians. Since the health professional is key in transmitting information to people, resolving skepticism, and increasing confidence in science and vaccines, effective strategies must be disseminated to the professionals.

4.3.2 Community Engagement

In addition to improving communication, strong community engagement is a valuable strategy to overcome vaccine hesitancy. This involves engaging community members, such as health workers, religious leaders, barbers, and teachers, to provide accurate and culturally relevant information about vaccines and to address common concerns and myths. For example, a study in Maryland found that conversations between barbers and their clients increased vaccine acceptance among Black men [24].

Community engagement is critical in developing countries where it is challenging to reach low-income and underserved communities for vaccine coverage. Personalized information campaigns and community mobilization can aid in vaccine uptake. This can include building awareness campaigns in public places such as shops, markets, and places of worship. Community leaders (religious and political) can help spread awareness about vaccinations. This was demonstrated recently in Pakistan to promote COVID-19 vaccine coverage [25]. Another study in India found that community healthcare professionals and medical interns improved vaccine coverage (universally recommended vaccines for children, adolescents, and adults) among rural populations by conducting home visits, group meetings, and educational sessions [26].

Vaccine uptake, however, depends on vaccination access [25]. In some remote locations that do not have access to vaccination sites, mobile vaccination camps can help provide access to vaccines. Such camps can be organized in collaboration with local community-based organizations and nongovernmental organizations (NGOs). The mobile camps serve as a place to assemble people, counsel them, and register them for vaccination. This was demonstrated in the study conducted in regions of Pakistan during the COVID-19 vaccine campaign. The study raised awareness and removed vaccine access barriers through community mobilization. The outcome showed that interventions in some low-income and underserved communities helped improve willingness to vaccinate by 7% and vaccine uptake by 17%. The study further demonstrated that vaccine awareness increased and hesitancy decreased following the awareness interventions.

Similarly, a study conducted on childhood immunization services in Sierra Leone following the 2014–2016 Ebola epidemic showed that community engagement correlated strongly with confidence in vaccination and its uptake [27]. This study highlighted the program in Sierra Leone, where a civil society platform exists to strengthen community engagement in delivering childhood immunizations. In this location, outcomes of interest were measured by conducting household surveys by engaging multiple participants. These platforms must include community-based organizations, nongovernmental organizations (local and international), teacher's associations, physician associations, and local news media organizations. Such strategies help bring together important community stakeholders, and the programs can be built in individual locations based on local needs.

All these studies note that there is no one-size-fits-all approach to community engagement. This makes it difficult to evaluate and compare the effect of community engagement across countries. In 2020, UNICEF developed a set of minimum quality standards for community engagement that can guide the development and evaluation of community engagement interventions [28].

4.3.3 Monetary Incentives

One strategy to increase the uptake of vaccines is to use money to motivate the public to get vaccinated. However, this method is controversial and has had mixed results in studies, many of which have not been randomized trials. One randomized study that tested the efficacy of this method showed that money could increase vaccine participation by about four percentage points [29]. The study conducted in Sweden preregistered approximately 8000 participants for a COVID-19 vaccine. The study showed that a modest payment of 24 U.S. dollars (200 Swedish Kronor) increased vaccination rates by 4.2 percentage points ($P = 0.005$) from a baseline rate of 71.6%.

In the United States, in response to the 1989–1991 measles epidemic, congress passed the Omnibus Budget Reconciliation Act (OBRA) on August 10, 1993, and created the Vaccines for Children (VFC) Program, which provides vaccines to children whose parents or guardians may not be able to afford them [57]. The VFC Program became operational on October 1, 1994. Section 1928 of the Social Security Act is an entitlement program (a right granted by law) for eligible children ages 18 and younger. The program was designed to improve vaccine availability nationwide by providing vaccines at no cost to VFC Program-eligible children through VFC program-enrolled public and private healthcare providers. The Office of Management and Budget (OMB) approves funding for the VFC Program and then allocates the funds through the Centers for Medicare & Medicaid Services (CMS) to the CDC. After receiving the funds, the CDC buys the vaccines at a discount and distributes them to VFC Program providers at the direction of awardees (i.e., the 61 state, local, and territorial immunization programs that receive operational funding from the CDC to implement and oversee their VFC Programs).

Before using COVID-19 vaccines, incentive-based approaches mainly involved childhood vaccinations in rural and lower socioeconomic areas. For example, a study in Pakistan found that giving cash transfers to low-income families increased the demand for childhood immunization by 12 percentage points [26]. In contrast, a study in the United States during the COVID-19 pandemic showed that monetary rewards were ineffective in some populations who remained hesitant and refused to get vaccinated. In scenarios where it may have worked, giving gifts over lotteries was a more successful approach. The study showed that an alternative approach, such as imposing costs on those hesitant to vaccinate, was generally more effective. The costs involved higher health insurance premiums or job loss at times [30].

Another unique strategy to promote influenza vaccination among children and people over 60 years old was studied in China. The study examined how a pay-it-forward intervention compared to the standard of care user-paid vaccination system. The pay-it-forward intervention consisted of a free influenza vaccine and an opportunity to donate financially to support the vaccination of other individuals. The study showed that 107 (96%) of 111 participants in the pay-it-forward group donated money for subsequent vaccinations. The pay-it-forward group had a lower economic cost (calculated as the cost without subtraction of donations) per person vaccinated (U.S. $45·60) than did the standard-of-care group ($64·67). Additionally, the vaccination rate in the pay-it-forward group was also higher than the rate in the non-pay-it-forward groups [31].

In the United States, a study assessed the impact of categories of interventions on people's willingness to be vaccinated against influenza [32]. This study showed that having easy access to drop-in vaccination sites was important in all age groups (18–40, 41–64, and 65 years and above). Small financial incentives contributed to high vaccine willingness in the younger age group (18–40). The study also noted that recommendations from clinicians were the most influential driver of vaccine willingness over any other sources, and this is consistent with other studies that concluded similarly.

The recent COVID-19 pandemic highlighted the stumbling blocks that impact vaccination uptake. Governments and businesses have attempted to incentivize vaccine uptake or impose disincentives for vaccine refusal. In the United States, in 2021, Ohio created a $1 million lottery for randomly selected vaccine recipients. In 2022, in the province of Quebec, to enter locations where alcohol and cannabis were sold, people needed a vaccine passport. Analyses of the two methodologies implemented showed that the impact on vaccine adoption was minimal at best following the Ohio lottery [33, 34]. In contrast, after the announcement by Québec Health Minister Christian Dubé, daily appointments for the first doses of COVID-19 vaccines in Quebec quadrupled in anticipation of the liquor and cannabis stores' restriction deadline [35].

Concerning COVID-19, it was observed that monetary incentives have remained controversial in their ability to improve vaccine uptake. Mandatory COVID-19 certification to access public venues, workplaces, and nonessential businesses met with some success, but such programs must be designed carefully. Much research suggests that motivation derived from losses is more significant than that obtained from comparable gains [36–38].

4.3.4 Use of Technology

In an era of pervasive use of technology, a wise move would be to harness technology to aid in vaccine information distribution. Vaccination strategies, including identifying at-risk patients, engaging community partners and locations, and providing in-person education or assistance, should be combined with health information technology to improve vaccination efforts [58]. There are pros and cons associated with the wide use of technology, especially to ensure scientifically accurate information is being disseminated to the public. Strategies must be applied to help increase vaccine adoption, dispel inaccuracy and misinformation, amplify communication from trusted sources and subject matter experts, and monitor information spread.

Many strategies have included reminder phone calls to people, text messages, and emails. Studies have shown that simple recall messages via short message service (SMS) were preferred; however, their effectiveness is less clear. Such strategies have also used informative posters, leaflets, videotapes, graphs, charts, animated images, social media, lectures, etc. As we learn where and how people obtain their healthcare information, vaccine messaging must be adjusted to reflect modern practices. Harnessing the internet and social media can deliver the message about vaccines to many people.

Innovative use of technology to improve vaccine uptake has involved using film to deliver vaccine information. In Northern Nigeria, in an attempt to break community barriers to polio vaccination, a campaign called "Majigi" was designed [39]. In the native Hausa language, Majigi denoted a roadside film show conducted in communities by mobile vans. The pilot campaign included a series of polio video clips that dealt with the known misconceptions about polio in the selected settlements, including the belief that an evil spirit or demon caused the disease. Majigi educational intervention targeted the beliefs about the cause of polio disease and the negative attitude toward polio vaccination as two important and changeable factors for the very low uptake of polio vaccination in these communities.

Before the Majigi campaign, regular polio supplemental vaccination activities were conducted in November 2008, and the uptake in these settlements was documented. After the Majigi awareness campaign, monthly supplemental regular vaccination activities were monitored for six months, and cumulative uptake in each settlement was documented. Results showed an upward trend in the uptake of polio vaccination in all the settlements after the introduction of the Majigi campaign. The consistent increase in vaccinated children and the cumulative coverage was four times greater than the value observed with only regular supplemental vaccination activities before the introduction of Majigi. This suggested a change in the attitude of the targeted communities toward polio vaccination and decreased community rejection of routine polio vaccination activities.

Since the COVID-19 pandemic, many studies have shown that people can easily access health-related information on social media platforms. While social media is often used to share personalized and culturally relevant content, there is a question about the accuracy of the information. However, it could have a positive impact if the information presented is culturally tailored health messaging through trusted sources (health professionals, public health agencies) [40]. This must involve communities in developing relevant specific messages and approaches. Moreover, it should support community-driven initiatives to identify at-risk groups, find and work with local influencers, and define meaningful content for communication campaigns. Social media platform companies should exercise more accountability and sign pledges to systematically track and remove harmful content that undermines public health measures, particularly during a public health crisis. The message must also avoid being a narrow focus and instead strive to be a two-way street to learn the misconceptions and how to improve upon those. The public must be empowered to identify and flag misinformation on social media. Information presented on these platforms must also be systematically monitored, and there must be timely rebuttal of misinformation from trusted health professionals. While there has been some backlash against government agencies influencing social media platforms to manage misinformation, there may be an opportunity for influential physician groups and other professional bodies to approach social media platforms with a case for managing misinformation.

Social media can also be harnessed as a tool to measure vaccination uptake. In the United States to monitor influenza vaccine uptake, there are two national surveillance systems: the CDC FluVax view, which assembles uptake data from several national surveys, and the national vaccine program office, which uses an online tool to track influenza vaccination insurance claims from Medicare users [41, 42]. Surveillance data is usually collected on a monthly or yearly basis. However, with social media platforms like X (i.e., formerly known as Twitter), data can be obtained weekly [43]. The robustness of the tools used to mine these platforms must be fine-tuned to remove noise or excess unrelated information and obtain uniform information across different locations. The ability to integrate these novel methods into existing frameworks and validate new data streams against reliable metrics will help us progress in a new direction.

Studies that have looked at social media platforms such as Reddit note that interventions designed to employ these mediums must consider the cultures of the online community [44]. This will ensure members on the platform absorb the information from the campaign effectively. Policymakers should work with individuals who can provide support on these platforms and can actively maintain an online community to facilitate the intervention. Research has shown that the most successful interventions delivered using technology, especially those that involve the use of the Web, are interactive with the user. In addition, when the information is presented as a narrative, there is more success in its acceptability and effectiveness [45]. Information presented on webpages as a narrative is gauged as being user-friendly and allows the users to decide the plot's direction and determine the vaccination's necessity.

Evidence has shown that the increasing use of technology and especially reliance on the use of online content has contributed to the spread of vaccine misinformation and vaccine hesitancy [59]. However, with the use of technologies like artificial intelligence (AI), an artificial intelligence-generated promotion of vaccines can help minimize hesitancy and be used to drive vaccine uptake.

AI and associated technologies are increasingly being applied in the healthcare sector. Healthcare professionals and organizations have started to discuss incorporating AI, machine learning, and deep learning into their practices to deliver care [60]. In recent years, deep learning has been widely used in primary health care. For example, diabetic retinopathy in healthcare centers can be detected by an AI system developed by Abramoff et al. and approved by the Federal Drug Administration of the USA [61]. Machine learning methods were also used in the health sector by [62] to identify children at risk of not being vaccinated against Measles, Mumps, and Rubella in WHO countries. Through the use of the AI-generated chatbot, the message generated in favor of an evidence-based approach and opting to follow scientific discoveries rather than myths could be a possible way to reduce vaccine hesitancy as well as similar tendencies in future pandemics [63]. Factors that may contribute to the effectiveness of vaccine chatbots include their ability to provide credible and personalized information in real-time, as well as the familiarity and accessibility of the chatbot platform to users.

Novel technologies such as Large Language Models (LLMs) are AI designed to reproduce human language processing capabilities. They use deep learning techniques, such as artificial neural networks, and can learn and process large amounts of language data from various sources. [64]. LLMs have also generated interest among healthcare professionals, considering their potential to improve health and patients' lives. These tools could help physicians process the growing amount of medical data and complexity of clinical decisions, make timely, informed decisions, and improve the overall quality/efficiency of healthcare. Such technologies can also be used to study people's behaviors and attitudes. They could be a valuable tool to help public health authorities guide vaccination policies, design new health education, and continue information interventions aimed at the public.

However, before implementing these approaches in policy, issues related to AI require more research. External validation, integration into a medical roadmap, and support from clinicians are needed to adopt them. There are also ethical and implementation concerns in AI applications, including data issues in the training and AI hallucinations. Moreover, the dependence on AI changes the patient–clinician relation dynamics. Therefore, appropriate collective knowledge regarding AI is required to help healthcare professionals, organizations, and departments decide how to use AI systems.

4.4 How Do We Evaluate Active Learning Sessions for Their Efficacy?

Effective implementation of immunization programs must rely on a multi-pronged approach involving clinician/patient/involvement, good communication, use of technology, and community-based engagement. Strategies used to improve vaccine uptake can target one or, ideally, all groups involved in achieving the goal. Often, the primary outcome of a strategy employed is the measure of vaccination rates (vaccine uptake or vaccine coverage). Given the many influencers of vaccine uptake, a better assessment of vaccine uptake strategies should consider secondary outcomes, including willingness to receive immunization, access to healthcare for immunization-related issues, attitudes/perceptions/knowledge toward vaccination, and perceived helpfulness/rate of use of the intervention. Information on these parameters can be obtained through electronic surveys, polls, household surveys, telephone surveys, and physician meeting sessions.

It has been shown that vaccine literacy is crucial to overcoming vaccine hesitancy and improving vaccine uptake. Vaccine literacy is defined as the ability of people to access, process, and understand basic vaccination knowledge and vaccination services, as well as to assess the potential consequences and risks of their behavior and make health-related decisions [46]. While vaccine literacy is important, it has been indicated that tools used to assess it are inadequate and merely adopted from health literacy studies. Since the COVID-19 pandemic, there has been a push to develop better tools to assess vaccine literacy; this incorporates measuring health literacy skills and includes items for evaluating outcomes, such as attitudes, beliefs, and behaviors that impact vaccine uptake.

Conducting audits and feedback is an effective strategy for improving immunization practices. The state of Georgia's health department developed a program called Assessment, Feedback, Incentives, and Exchange (AFIX), which was then expanded by the CDC. This program is now used widely across the United States. It has been shown to be effective in increasing childhood immunization rates following its implementation in public clinics and private practices [47, 48]. AFIX uses clinic-level audits and feedback to providers.

One of the strengths of using active learning strategies to influence vaccine uptake is the ability to cater the programs specifically to the location and specific target audience. However, because of the variation in the types of strategies employed, determining the strategy's success is often difficult. The WHO Working Group on the Behavioral and Social Drivers of Vaccination is developing standardized quantitative and qualitative tools to help measure behavioral and social drivers of vaccination. These tools will help understand what drives the uptake of vaccines. It is intended for immunization program managers and others who collect, analyze, and use the data for vaccine program planning and evaluation. The drivers that are measured include beliefs and experiences specific to vaccination. The tool focuses on measurable factors in individuals and can be tailored to the particular vaccination program. It does not directly include broader factors such as literacy, political views, and socioeconomic status; these can be explored using the program's qualitative tools. Routine tracking of the collected data will offer insights into how to improve program implementation continually [49].

Here are some examples of active learning strategies that can help increase the uptake of vaccines. Interventions that can improve uptake are multicomponent and should focus on dialogue-based approaches. They should target multiple audiences and consider social aspects to achieve positive results. It is also essential to build trust and rapport with the audience and communicate with empathy and respect. Strategies should involve people from the community and must employ good communication among all concerned parties. However, it is essential to note that different strategies (such as monetary incentives or the use of technology) may work better for different audiences and contexts, depending on their needs, preferences, and barriers. Vaccine hesitancy, awareness, and knowledge must be addressed at the community and social network level, not just at the individual level. Therefore, it is advisable to tailor the intervention strategies to each group's specific characteristics and concerns, develop culturally sensitive programming and materials, and evaluate their effectiveness using appropriate methods.

Key Takeaways

It is important to recognize the significance of vaccine literacy, conduct audits and feedback to improve immunization practices, and employ active learning strategies to increase vaccine uptake. There is no one-size-fits-all approach to improving vaccine uptake, and different methods may be required depending on the context and audience. Therefore, it is crucial to tailor intervention strategies to the specific characteristics and concerns of each group and evaluate their effectiveness using appropriate methods.

It is essential to emphasize the role of communication from trusted sources to address vaccine hesitancy, awareness, and knowledge in communities. A collaborative approach that involves people from the community and employs good communication among all concerned parties is necessary to achieve positive results.

Therefore, building trust and rapport with the audience and communicating with empathy and respect is crucial. By doing so, we can work together to increase vaccine uptake and promote public health.

An additional important factor in improving vaccine uptake is access to vaccines. Factors that affect vaccine hesitancy also affect vaccine access. Both access and hesitancy are related in complex ways to social determinants of health. Vaccine access and hesitancy barriers must be addressed through local communication campaigns and vaccination programs that deliver and administer vaccines at patients' homes or places of work. The United States, the United Kingdom, and other countries are working to take the lessons learned from the last few years to drive policy toward advancing vaccine equity [64–67]. Such policies can help change clinician practices and individual patients' behavior and help increase vaccine uptake.

References

1. World Health Organization Strategic Advisory Group of Experts (SAGE) on immunization: report of the SAGE Working Group on Vaccine Hesitancy. 2014.
2. Kestenbaum LA, Feemster KA. Identifying and addressing vaccine hesitancy. Pediatr Ann. 2015;44:e71–5. PMID: 25875982; PMCID: PMC4475845
3. Pitts PJ, Poland GA. Trust and science: public health's home field advantage in addressing vaccine hesitancy and improving immunization rates. Vaccine. 2023;41(38):5483–5., ISSN 0264-410X. https://doi.org/10.1016/j.vaccine.2023.08.003.
4. Kelley MS, Su D, Britigan DH. Disparities in health information access: results of a county-wide survey and implications for health communication. Health Commun. 2016;31(5):575–82.
5. Poínhos R, Oliveira BM, van der Lans IA, Fischer AR, Berezowska A, Rankin A, et al. Providing personalized nutrition: consumers' trust and preferences regarding sources of information, service providers and regulators, and communication channels. Public Health Genomics. 2017;20:218.
6. Privor-Dumm L, Excler J, Gilbert S, et al. Vaccine access, equity, and justice: COVID-19 vaccines and vaccination. BMJ Glob Health. 2023;8:e011881.
7. European Centre for Disease Prevention and Control. Catalogue of interventions addressing vaccine hesitancy. Stockholm: ECDC; 2017.
8. Jarrett C, Wilson R, O'Leary M, Eckersberger E, Larson HJ. Strategies for addressing vaccine hesitancy—a systematic review. Vaccine. 2015;33:4180–90.
9. Dubé E, Gagnon D, MacDonald NE. Strategies intended to address vaccine hesitancy: review of published reviews. Vaccine. 2015;33:4191–203.
10. Stitzer ML, Polk T, Bowles S, Kosten T. Drug users' adherence to a 6-month vaccination protocol: effects of motivational incentives. Drug Alcohol Depend. 2010;107(1):76–9.
11. LaMontagne DS, Barge S, Le NT, Mugisha E, Penny ME, Gandhi S, et al. Human papillomavirus vaccine delivery strategies that achieved high coverage in low- and middle-income countries. Bull World Health Organ. 2011;89(11):821.
12. Wang L, Li J, Chen H, Li F, Armstrong GL, Nelson C, et al. Hepatitis B vaccination of newborn infants in rural China: evaluation of a village-based, out-of-cold-chain delivery strategy. Bull World Health Organ. 2007;85(9):688–94.
13. Al-Tawil MM, El-Gohary EE, El-Sayed MH. Effect of infection control strategy on knowledge, attitude and practice towards hepatitis B transmission and prevention in vulnerable populations. Int J Risk Saf Med. 2013;25(3):135–43.

14. Harris K, Maurer J, Black C, Euler G, Kadiyala S. Workplace efforts to promote influenza vaccination among healthcare personnel and their association with uptake during the 2009 pandemic influenza A (H1N1). Vaccine. 2011;29(16):2978–85.
15. Kondji D. Synthesis of the major realizations of EPI communication for West and Central Francophone African Countries. The Communication Initiative; 2006.
16. Office of the Surgeon General (OSG). Confronting health misinformation: the U.S. Surgeon General's Advisory on Building a Healthy Information Environment [Internet]. Washington (DC): US Department of Health and Human Services; 2021. PMID: 34283416. https://www.ncbi.nlm.nih.gov/books/NBK572168/
17. Tuckerman J, Kaufman J, Danchin M. Effective approaches to combat vaccine hesitancy. Pediatr Infect Dis J. 2022;41(5):e243–5. https://doi.org/10.1097/INF.0000000000003499.
18. Ryan J, Malinga T. Interventions for vaccine hesitancy. Curr Opin Immunol. 2021;71:89–91.
19. Dubé E, Gagnon D, Vivion M. Optimizing communication material to address vaccine hesitancy. Can Commun Dis Rep. 2020;46(2/3):48–52. https://doi.org/10.14745/ccdr.v46i23a05.
20. Gagneur A, Dubé È, Farrands A, Lemaître T, Boulianne N, Sauvageau C, et al. Promoting vaccination at birth with motivational interviewing session improves vaccination intention and reduces vaccine hesitancy. E-Poster presentation. Brighton: 2016, May. 34th annual meeting of the European society for pediatric infectious diseases (ESPID); 2016.
21. Dempsey AF, Pyrznawoski J, Lockhart S, Barnard J, Campagna EJ, Garrett K, et al. Effect of a health care professional communication training intervention on adolescent human papillomavirus vaccination: a cluster randomized clinical trial. JAMA Pediatr. 2018:E180016.
22. Brewer NT, Hall ME, Malo TL, et al. Announcements versus conversations to improve HPV vaccination coverage: a randomized trial. Pediatrics. 2017;139:e20161764.
23. Anderson KM, Leister S, De Rego R. The 5Ts for Teach Back: An Operational Definition for Teach-Back Training. Health Lit Res Pract. 2020;4(2):e94–e103. https://doi.org/10.3928/24748307-20200318-01. PMID: 32293689; PMCID: PMC7156258.
24. Lowry M, Shefska D. Fighting vaccine hesitancy: what can we learn from social science? National Academies July 1; 2021. https://www.nationalacademies.org/news/2021/07/fighting-vaccine-hesitancy-what-can-we-learn-from-social-science
25. Abdullah M, Ahmad T, Kazmi T, Sultan F, Afzal S, Safdar RM, Khan AA. Community engagement to increase vaccine uptake: quasi-experimental evidence from Islamabad and Rawalpindi, Pakistan. PloS one. 2022;17(12):e0274718. https://doi.org/10.1371/journal.pone.0274718.
26. Singh P, Dhalaria P, Kashyap S, et al. Strategies to overcome vaccine hesitancy: a systematic review. Syst Rev. 2022;11:78. https://doi.org/10.1186/s13643-022-01941-4.
27. Jalloh MF, Sengeh P, Ibrahim N, Kulkarni S, Sesay T, Eboh V, Jalloh MB, Abu Pratt S, Webber N, Thomas H, Kaiser R, Singh T, Prybylski D, Omer SB, Brewer NT, Wallace AS. Association of community engagement with vaccination confidence and uptake: a cross-sectional survey in Sierra Leone, 2019. J Glob Health. 2022;12:04006. https://doi.org/10.7189/jogh.12.04006.
28. UNICEF. Minimum quality standards and indicators in community engagement. 2020. https://www.unicef.org/mena/reports/community-engagement-standards. Accessed 1 Aug 2020.
29. Campos-Mercade P, Meier AN, Schneider FH, Meier S, Pope D, Wengström E. Monetary incentives increase COVID-19 vaccinations. Science (New York). 2021;374(6569):879–82. https://doi.org/10.1126/science.abm0475.
30. Bennett NG, Bloom DE, Ferranna M. Factors underlying COVID-19 vaccine and booster hesitancy and refusal, and incentivizing vaccine adoption. PLoS One. 2022;17(9):e0274529. https://doi.org/10.1371/journal.pone.0274529.
31. Wu D, et al. Effectiveness of a pay-it-forward intervention compared with user-paid vaccination to improve influenza vaccine uptake and community engagement among children and older adults in China: a quasi-experimental pragmatic trial. Lancet Infect Dis. 2022;22(10):1484–92. https://doi.org/10.1016/S1473-3099(22)00346-2.

32. Bonner KE, Chyderiotis S, Sicsic J, Mueller JE, Ulrich AK, Toomey T, Horvath KJ, Neaton JD, Basta NE. What motivates adults to accept influenza vaccine? An assessment of incentives, ease of access, messaging, and sources of information using a discrete choice experiment. SSM—population health. 2023;22:101384. https://doi.org/10.1016/j.ssmph.2023.101384.
33. Barber A, West J. Conditional cash lotteries increase COVID-19 vaccination rates. J Health Econ [Internet]. 2022;81:102578. https://linkinghub.elsevier.com/retrieve/pii/S0167629621001636. pmid:34986437
34. Walkey AJ, Law A, Bosch NA. Lottery-based incentive in Ohio, and COVID-19 vaccination rates. JAMA [Internet]. 2021;326(8):766. https://jamanetwork.com/journals/jama/fullarticle/2781792. pmid:34213530
35. The Canadian Press. First-dose vaccinations quadruple in Quebec ahead of restrictions at liquor and cannabis stores. 2022. https://montreal.ctvnews.ca/first-dose-vaccinations-quadruple-in-quebec-ahead-of-restrictions-at-liquor-and-cannabis-stores-1.5731327
36. Karaivanov A, Kim D, Lu SE, Shigeoka H. COVID-19 vaccination mandates and vaccine uptake. NBER Work Pap Ser [Internet]; 2021. p. 29563. http://www.nber.org/papers/w29563.pdf
37. Mills MC, Rüttenauer T. The effect of mandatory COVID-19 certificates on vaccine uptake: synthetic-control modeling of six countries. Lancet Public Heal [Internet]. 2022;7(1):e15–22. https://linkinghub.elsevier.com/retrieve/pii/S2468266721002735. pmid:34914925
38. Kahneman D, Tversky A. Prospect theory: an analysis of decision under risk. Econometrica [Internet]. 1979;47(2):263. https://www.jstor.org/stable/1914185?origin=crossref
39. Nasiru SG, Aliyu GG, Gasasira A, Aliyu MH, Zubair M, Mandawari SU, et al. Breaking community barriers to polio vaccination in Northern Nigeria: the impact of a grassroots mobilization campaign (Majigi). Pathog Glob Health. 2012;106(3):166–71. https://doi.org/10.1179/2047773212Y.0000000018.
40. Goldsmith LP, Rowland-Pomp M, Hanson K, Deal A, Crawshaw AF, Hayward SE, Knights F, Carter J, Ahmad A, Razai M, Vandrevala T, Hargreaves S. Use of social media platforms by migrant and ethnic minority populations during the COVID-19 pandemic: a systematic review. BMJ Open. 2022;12(11):e061896. https://doi.org/10.1136/bmjopen-2022-061896.
41. Centers for Disease Control and Prevention. Influenza Vaccination Coverage | FluVaxView | Seasonal Influenza | CDC. 2017. https://www.cdc.gov/flu/fluvaxview/index.htm. Accessed 18 Sept 2023.
42. US Department of Health and Human Services. Flu vaccination trends. 2017. https://www.hhs.gov/nvpo/resources/flu/index.html
43. Huang X, Smith MC, Jamison AM, Broniatowski DA, Dredze M, Quinn SC, Cai J, Paul MJ. Can online self-reports assist in real-time identification of influenza vaccination uptake? A cross-sectional study of influenza vaccine-related tweets in the USA, 2013–2017. BMJ Open. 2019;9(1):e024018. https://doi.org/10.1136/bmjopen-2018-024018.
44. Sun Y, Hamedani MF, Javidi G, Sheybani E, Hao F. Examining COVID-19 vaccine attitude using SEM-artificial neural networks approach: a case from Reddit community. Health Promot Int. 2022;37(6):daac157. https://doi.org/10.1093/heapro/daac157.
45. Wang Q, Zhang W. The use of Web-based interactive technology to promote HPV vaccine uptake among young females: a randomized controlled trial. BMC Womens Health. 2021;21(1):277. https://doi.org/10.1186/s12905-021-01417-y.
46. Zhang E, Dai Z, Wang S, Wang X, Zhang X, Fang Q. Vaccine literacy and vaccination: a systematic review. Int J Public Health. 2023;68:1605606. https://doi.org/10.3389/ijph.2023.1605606.
47. LeBaron CW, Mercer JT, Massoudi MS, et al. Changes in clinic vaccination coverage after institution of measurement and feedback in 4 states and two cities. Arch Pediatr Adolesc Med. 1999;153:879–86.
48. Massoudi MS, Walsh J, Stokley S, et al. Assessing immunization performance of private practitioners in Maine: impact of the assessment, feedback, incentives, and exchange strategy. Pediatrics. 1999;103:1218–23.

49. World Health Organization. Behavioral and social drivers of vaccination: tools and practical guidance for achieving high uptake. Geneva; 2022. License: CC BY-NC-SA 3.0 IGO
50. Hornsey MJ, Harris EA, Fielding KS. The psychological roots of anti-vaccination attitudes: a 24-nation investigation. Health Psychol. 2018;37:307–15. https://doi.org/10.1037/hea0000586.
51. European Centre for Disease Prevention and Control. Accessed Sept 2023. https://www.ecdc.europa.eu/en/news-events/e-learning-understanding-vaccine-acceptance-strategies-increase-vaccine-uptake
52. CITI Program. Accessed Sept 2023. https://about.citiprogram.org/course/communicating-research-findings/.
53. Center for Disease Control. Accessed Sept 2023. https://www.cdc.gov/vaccines/ed/youcalltheshots.html
54. Stephens AB, Hofstetter AM, Stockwell MS. Influenza vaccine hesitancy: scope, influencing factors, and strategic interventions. Pediatr Clin N Am. 2023;70(2):227–41. https://doi.org/10.1016/j.pcl.2022.11.003.
55. Galagali PM, Kinikar AA, Kumar VS. Vaccine hesitancy: obstacles and challenges. Curr Pediatr Rep. 2022;10(4):241–8. https://doi.org/10.1007/s40124-022-00278-9.
56. Prescott WA Jr, Bernhardi C. Immunization education in US pharmacy colleges and schools. Am J Pharm Educ. 2019;83(5):6765. https://doi.org/10.5688/ajpe6765.
57. Vaccine for Children Program. (n.d.). https://www.cdc.gov/vaccines/programs/vfc/about/index.html
58. Prescott GM, Prescott WA. Health information technology utilization and impact on COVID-19 vaccination. J Am Pharm Assoc. 2021;61(4):e230–2., ISSN 1544-3191. https://doi.org/10.1016/j.japh.2021.03.020.
59. Rutten LJF, Zhu X, Leppin AL, Ridgeway JL, Swift MD, Griffin JM, Jacobson RM, et al. Evidence-based strategies for clinical organizations to address COVID-19 vaccine hesitancy. Mayo Clin Proc. 2021;96(3):699–707.
60. Miotto R, Wang F, Wang S, Jiang X, Dudley JT. Deep learning for healthcare: review, opportunities and challenges. Brief Bioinform. 2018;19(6):1236–46. https://doi.org/10.1093/bib/bbx044.
61. Abràmoff MD, Lavin PT, Birch M, Shah N, Folk JC. Pivotal trial of an autonomous AI-based diagnostic system for detection of diabetic retinopathy in primary care offices. NPJ Digit Med. 2018;1:39.
62. Bell A, Rich A, Teng M, et al. Proactive advising: a machine learning driven approach to vaccine hesitancy. 2019 IEEE International Conference on Healthcare Informatics (ICHI); 2019. p. 1–6. https://doi.org/10.1109/ICHI.2019.8904616.
63. Sohail SS, Madsen DØ, Farhat F, et al. ChatGPT and vaccines: can AI Chatbots boost awareness and uptake? Ann Biomed Eng. 2024;52:446–50. https://doi.org/10.1007/s10439-023-03305-y.
64. Deiana G, Dettori M, Arghittu A, Azara A, Gabutti G, Castiglia P. Artificial intelligence and public health: evaluating ChatGPT responses to vaccination myths and misconceptions. Vaccine. 2023;11:1217. https://doi.org/10.3390/vaccines11071217.
65. Essien UR, Dusetzina SB. Cost-related barriers and ensuring equitable access to vaccines in the US. JAMA Pediatr. 2023;177(11):1117–8. https://doi.org/10.1001/jamapediatrics.2023.3260.
66. London D. Evidence review for interventions to increase the uptake of routine vaccines by improving access: Vaccine uptake in the general population: National Institute for Health and Care Excellence (NICE). (NICE Guideline, No. 218); 2022 May. https://www.ncbi.nlm.nih.gov/books/NBK581887/
67. Kathryn M., Anderson Sarah, Leister Ruth, De Rego (2020) The 5Ts for Teach Back: An Operational Definition for Teach-Back Training HLRP: Health Literacy Research and Practice 4(2) https://doi.org/10.3928/24748307-20200318-01

Chapter 5
Vaccine Education: From Foundations to Clinical Application

Michelle L. Demory and Amanda J. Chase

5.1 Introduction

In 2019, with an exponential rise in vaccine-preventable illnesses, the World Health Organization identified vaccine hesitancy as a top-ten threat to global health [1]. Vaccine hesitancy is defined as delay or refusal of vaccination despite vaccine availability. Reasons for vaccine hesitancy vary, particularly with respect to geographic location. For instance, in low-income countries, vaccine uptake rates are low due to a lack of access. However, in high-income countries like Europe and the United States where vaccines are more easily accessible, reasons for vaccine hesitancy appear to be more varied, yet tend to center on vaccine safety, usefulness, and efficacy [2].

Vaccine hesitancy was once thought to be a static state of vaccine refusal. However, more recent research suggests a swinging pendulum of hesitation toward vaccination [3]. One side represents refusal of all vaccinations, and the other side represents acceptance of all vaccinations without hesitation (Fig. 5.1). In the middle lies the selective delay of some or all vaccines or acceptance of some vaccines. Vaccine acceptance, delay, or refusal can all be influenced by the type of vaccine, risk, mistrust, access, and social factors [2].

Due to the global health concerns raised by a lack of vaccination and its association with misinformation and mistrust, healthcare providers play a pivotal role in helping patients understand the importance of vaccination and in refuting misinformation. Previous studies have shown the importance of taking a holistic and empathetic approach to having vaccine conversations with patients. Thus, it is crucial to

M. L. Demory (✉) · A. J. Chase
Department of Medical Education, Dr. Kiran C. Patel College of Allopathic Medicine, Nova Southeastern University, Fort Lauderdale, FL, USA
e-mail: Michelle.Demory@nova.edu

A. J. Chase et al. (eds.), *Vaccine Hesitancy Curriculum*,
https://doi.org/10.1007/978-3-031-88668-3_5

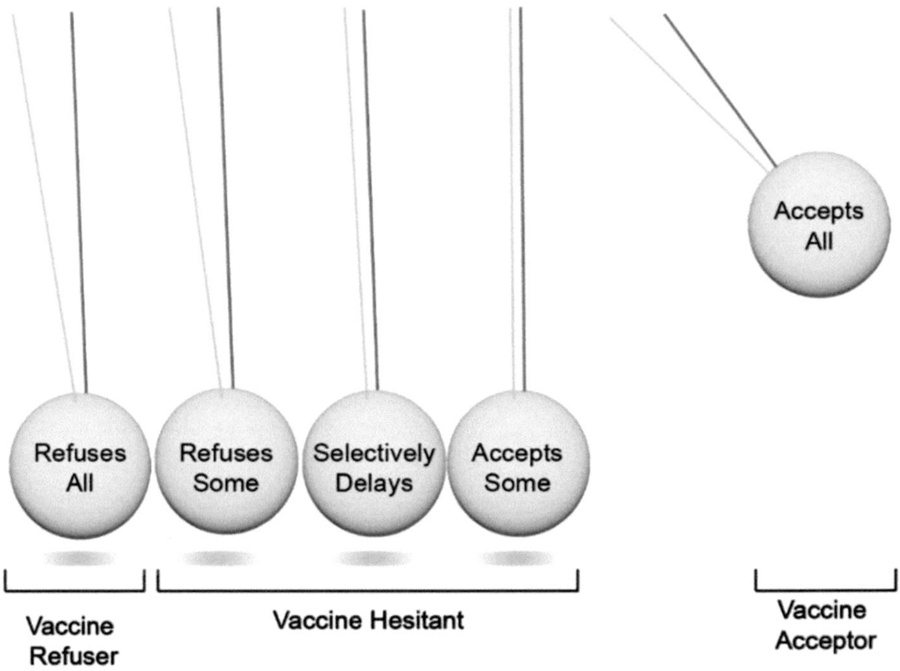

Fig. 5.1 Pendulum of vaccine hesitancy

aid health professions students not only in developing a strong foundational understanding of the history, pathophysiology, and ongoing research about vaccines but also in developing soft skills that are important to having productive controversial conversations with patients. Ideally, these will be developed and integrated at various points during graduate education, both in the foundational or preclinical curricula and during the applied or clinical curricula.

5.2 Section 1: Exploring Vaccine Curriculum

Vaccine education in the health professions encompasses not only the medical sciences basic to health professions but also an understanding of psychosocial determinants of health, best practices for recommending vaccination, and evidence-based communication strategies. Healthcare providers are often seen as the most trusted source of information regarding vaccination and training on how to approach vaccine communication with patients should be implemented early in health professions programs. Vaccine hesitancy educational tools for healthcare providers and trainees are predominantly centered around knowledge sharing and communication training [4]. These tools have been shown to create a positive impact on provider's self-perceived confidence in and likelihood of addressing vaccine-hesitant individuals. However, many of these existing curricular interventions are frequently facilitated as stand-alone sessions that lack integration within a longitudinal curricular theme. A recent study has underscored the paucity of experiential vaccine education sessions for health professions learners [5].

Integration of the foundational and applied sciences in health professions education promotes retention and application of the vast and ever-increasing wealth of knowledge [6]. Similarly, a vaccine education curriculum should be integrated across disciplines and clinical skills to emphasize the relevance of the sciences basic to medicine. When learned knowledge is required for engaging in decision-making or problem-solving, connected schemata, or memory structures, are created [6].

Cognitive integration is the creation of an integrated understanding of basic and clinical sciences within the mind of the learner [7]. For example, if learners are prompted to incorporate the science of vaccines into a role-play activity, they are integrating the communication skills with the sciences basic to medicine. Connected schemata, such as vaccine sciences and communication strategies are retrieved more efficiently from long-term memory when learners are confronted with scenarios in the workplace such as the patient–provider vaccine conversation. A study conducted by Schmidt et al. found that students exposed to active-learning, integrated curricula progress faster in problem-solving throughout their training when compared to traditional, didactic curricula [8]. In addition, we have previously shown that active-learning sessions on vaccine hesitancy topics help learners to integrate basic science, evidence-based studies, and clinical skills [9, 10].

5.2.1 Curriculum Design

Using the six-step curriculum design methodology popularized by Dr. David Kern in 1998, we have developed a multi-step, integrated vaccine education framework [11]. Backward design or the design of a curriculum with the outcomes in mind was at the core of our approach. Staying true to best practices in integrated session design, these vaccine education sessions integrate learning outcomes focused on knowledge, skills, and attitudes. Aligning with our previous experience in immunology and vaccine curriculum design at the medical, dental, and graduate school level, we believe vaccine education should incorporate evidence-based active learning approaches that focus on the development of vaccine knowledge and communication skills. The goal of the vaccine education curriculum is to cultivate communication skills in health professions trainees to dispel myths and disinformation, engender trust, and critically appraise the impact of health misinformation on patients and communities.

Each session within this framework seeks to complement health professions students' learning and experience levels, while also helping students develop their vaccine knowledge and skills such as communication, empathy, and professionalism. Assessment within the vaccine curriculum plays an essential role in the education of health professions learners by supporting each learner's understanding of their progress toward competencies in medical knowledge, interpersonal and communication skills, professionalism, and decision-making skills. Assessment outcomes should always be made available to provide learners with feedback on their performance and include suggestions for growth. Assessment of learning is typically divided into two types, summative and formative (Fig. 5.2). *Formative assessment* is an assessment *for learning*, and the purpose is to provide feedback that informs future learning and supports learners' understanding of their progressive development. Formative assessments should emphasize areas of strength, identify areas for improvement, and provide actionable feedback. Formative assessments are usually low stakes with little or no point value attached. They should be specific, timely, and frequent. *Summative assessment* is an assessment *of learning*, and the purpose is to deliver a judgment to improve learning and assess a learner's readiness to advance to the next phase of the curriculum. Summative assessments typically assign a grade to the learners' work and have a point value attached. Feedback from summative assessments should follow a rubric or detail the learner's achievement of the session learning objectives. Many programs will allow learners to watch a video of their performance and reflect on whether they planned appropriately for the assessment and how they can plan for future experiences.

The vaccine curriculum is learner-centered and integrates sessions on vaccine knowledge and communication skills. It consists of eight longitudinal sessions, is adaptable to any health professions program, and has the capacity to span anywhere from 1 year to 4 years of education (Fig. 5.3). The first four sessions are designed for implementation during the period in which the foundational sciences are emphasized, also referred to as the preclinical phase. The latter four sessions are designed for the period in which learners are focusing on the applied sciences, also referred to as the clinical phase. Each session builds upon the prior sessions, helping learners to integrate new knowledge with existing knowledge.

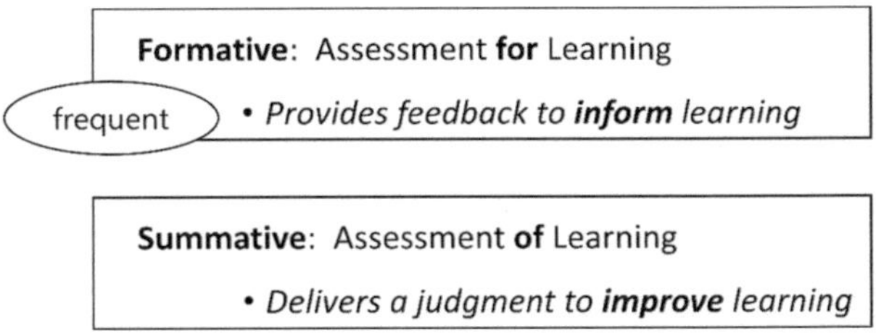

Fig. 5.2 Formative and summative assessment

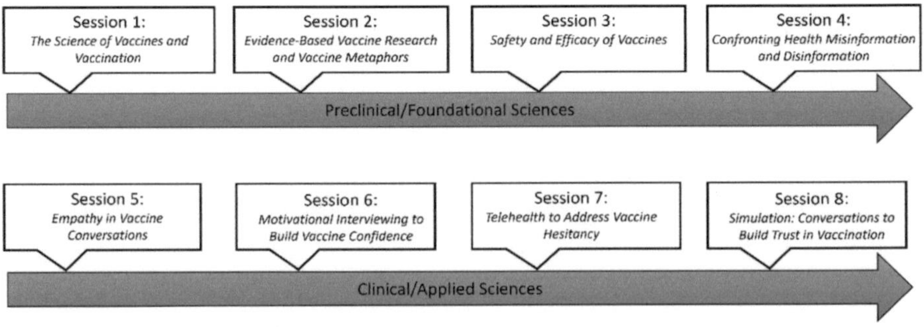

Fig. 5.3 Vaccine curriculum timeline

5.3 Section 2: Implementing Vaccine Curriculum

5.3.1 Session 1: The Science of Vaccines and Vaccination

5.3.1.1 Session 1 Rationale

Immunization has shaped modern medicine by protecting and promoting public health. Moreover, vaccines are attributed to increasing life expectancy by decreasing the morbidity and mortality associated with infectious diseases [12]. According to the CDC, more than 50 million deaths will be prevented by vaccination from 2021 to 2030 [13], with prevention of approximately four to five million deaths per year.

Clinicians play a fundamental role in maintaining high vaccination rates and are typically their patients' primary source for vaccine information. Therefore, understanding the purpose and underlying immune mechanisms of vaccination is crucial for health professions learners. While the topic of vaccines is traditionally taught during one or more didactic sessions, we believe that learners achieve longer-term recall and understanding when this material is reinforced in a flipped classroom, team-based learning style session.

5.3.1.2 Session 1 Overview

Learning outcomes	1. Compare and contrast active and passive immunization. 2. Distinguish between live attenuated and inactivated vaccines. 3. Discuss the host immune response to live attenuated and inactivated vaccines.
Format	Team-based learning
Duration	120 min

5.3.1.3 Session 1 Description

We recommend that this session be delivered early in the preclinical curriculum and should reinforce basic immunology and microbiology concepts. We suggest that the session be a two-hour team-based learning format [14]. Prereading should include textbook excerpts, review articles, or lectures. Readiness assurance test questions should address in multiple-choice format types of immunization (passive vs active), vaccines (attenuated vs inactivated), and basic immunology of the host response to vaccination. For the application activity, learners are placed into teams of 5–6. We propose the use of 3–4 clinical scenarios. Suggestions include: one case that focuses on passive immunization, with the possible use of Rh incompatibility or Zoster-immune globulin administration to an infant as examples; one case that compares and contrasts inactivated and live attenuated vaccines, with the possible use of oral polio vaccine and inactivated polio vaccine or intramuscular and intranasal influenza vaccines as examples; one case that evaluates post-vaccination symptomology (malaise, discomfort) and post-vaccination titer analyses as indicators for the immune response. Additional cases could focus on hypersensitivity reactions, vaccine and booster schedules, or infant vaccination.

5.3.1.4 Session 1 Evaluation

Formative assessment of higher-order thinking should be evaluated with the application activity. Summative assessment of basic concept pre-learning should be evaluated with the readiness assurance tests. Communication skills and teamwork can also be assessed by facilitator observation of team interactions.

5.3.2 Session 2: Evidence-Based Vaccine Research and Vaccine Metaphors

5.3.2.1 Session 2 Rationale

Healthcare practitioners should possess basic skills in critiquing the quality of evidence and assessing applicability to their patients. Underlying the skill set of practicing evidence-based medicine is the foundational knowledge an individual has and the self-awareness to identify gaps and fill them. To advance clinical effectiveness and evidence-based practice, the Institute of Medicine set a goal that by 2020, 90% of clinical decisions will be supported by accurate, timely, and up-to-date clinical information and will reflect the best available evidence to achieve the best patient outcomes. To incorporate the knowledge, skills, and attitudes required for evidence-based practice, many health professions programs interweave competencies and threads for evidence-based medicine into their curricula [15].

5.3.2.2 Session 2 Overview

Learning outcomes	1. Critically analyze the strengths and weaknesses of study designs, with special emphasis on the evaluation and interpretation of vaccine research. 2. Differentiate between myths and true contraindications to vaccination. 3. Utilize metaphors to communicate the risks and benefits of vaccination with a patient.
Format	Flipped classroom
Duration	120 min

5.3.2.3 Session 2 Description

The recommended format for a session on evidence-based vaccine research is a flipped classroom in which students are assigned research articles or reviews from the primary literature. To cultivate an understanding of the spectrum of vaccine hesitancy, it is important to introduce evidence-based literature from the vaccine research in addition to a weak, misinterpreted, or retracted study. In this session, we assign as pre-reading the since retracted Wakefield et al. manuscript [16] as an example of a research study that has since been disproved but is still exploited by antivaxxers to further their agenda. Within the 2 h large group session, first-year pharmacy and first-year medical students work in interprofessional small groups to analyze cohort studies that disprove the false hypothesis made by Andrew Wakefield. Debrief is a large group discussion about the learner groups' thoughts and findings. Subsequently, learner groups are prompted to practice communicating how vaccines work using vaccine metaphors and role-playing a patient encounter [9, 10].

5.3.2.4 Session 2 Evaluation

Formative assessment of communication skills following the vaccine conversation can occur through self and peer completion of a rubric. Learner engagement within the session is best evaluated using a survey instrument, called Assessing Student Perspective of Engagement in Class Tool (ASPECT), which comprehensively assesses the impact of the active-learning strategy [17].

5.3.3 Session 3: Safety and Efficacy of Vaccines

5.3.3.1 Session 3 Rationale

The recent resurgence of vaccine hesitancy during the COVID-19 pandemic once again brought to light adverse drug reactions associated with vaccination [18]. To better identify possible patient risks and to convey accurate information to patients, it is important for clinicians to understand vaccine formulations, components, myths related to these components, and true hypersensitivity reactions to vaccine components. This session is intended to be a fairly straightforward flipped-classroom style session to be delivered early in a health professions curriculum.

There are roughly six broad types of vaccines: inactivated, live attenuated, mRNA, viral vector, subunit/toxoid, and recombinant [19]. Each type is produced differently, includes different components, and induces different immune responses.

Common additional ingredients or components in vaccines are adjuvants, stabilizers, preservatives, and residual trace amounts of materials used during the production process. Collectively, these components are called excipients [20]. During development and FDA approval, vaccine formulations must undergo stringent testing in vitro, in vivo, and in human trials. As part of this process, all components of vaccines are safety tested, yet excipients are often a target of misinformation and misunderstanding.

Understanding the role of excipients, common myths surrounding them, and true hypersensitivity reactions to them is critical for clinicians in promoting vaccine efficacy and awareness [21–23]. This session is designed to address common patient concerns and provide practice for learners in how to respond to and discuss these concerns.

5.3.3.2 Session 3 Overview

Learning outcomes	1. Compare and contrast vaccine formulations. 2. Examine the active components, adjuvants, and excipients in vaccines and explain why they are present. 3. Address health misinformation according to vaccine ingredients and formulation. 4. Understand hypersensitivity reactions to vaccine components.
Format	Case-based learning
Duration	60 min

5.3.3.3 Session 3 Description

One week prior to the session, students are provided with the assigned reading, which details vaccine types and common components [20]. The run-time for this flipped classroom, case-based session is 60 min. Learners are placed into teams of approximately 4–5 for the first activity and in pairs for the second activity. For the first activity, learners are asked to list common excipients, to identify common myths and concerns surrounding excipients, and to discuss true hypersensitivity reactions to excipients as well as the underlying immune mechanisms. Poll Everywhere or other real-time response monitoring software is used during the debrief, with learner teams discussing their responses and facilitators providing clarification or explanation when needed.

For the second activity, learner pairs are asked to role-play in response to two sequentially released case scenarios. In the first scenario, a patient's mother expresses safety concerns over the presence of inactive ingredients, such as formaldehyde and aluminum. Learners are prompted to role-play, with one as the clinician and one as the mother. The learner clinician walks the mother through the ingredient list, using metaphors, to describe the necessity and safety of excipients. The learners are then asked to switch roles. In the second scenario, a healthy middle-age, previously vaccinated patient has a friend with a vaccine allergy. The patient is hesitant to receive booster vaccines because of his friend's experience. Learner pairs are prompted to role play, with the learner clinician walking the patient through allergic/hypersensitivity responses using metaphors and using empathetic communication to discuss the patient's vaccine history, vaccine components, and the risk of hypersensitivity reactions in a patient with no previous history. The learners are then asked to switch roles. During the debrief, learner pairs are asked to share the metaphors and communication strategies used in their simulated interaction.

5.3.3.4 Session 3 Evaluation

Formative assessment of communication skills during team activities and role-play scenarios can occur through self and peer completion of a rubric. Summative assessment could occur through a multiple choice-style assignment to be completed by teams during the first activity.

5.3.4 Session 4: Confronting Health Misinformation and Disinformation

5.3.4.1 Session 4 Rationale

The rapid propagation of misinformation and disinformation in the twenty-first century led to the coining of the term "infodemic" in 2003 [24]. A systematic review published in the Bulletin of the World Health Organization found that incorrect interpretations of health information led to increased vaccine hesitancy and delays in the provision of health care. Additionally, misleading and false health-related content led to mental, social, political, or economic distress. For these reasons, it is imperative that healthcare learners cultivate skills to confront misinformation and disinformation in patient–provider conversations.

5.3.4.2 Session 4 Overview

Learning outcomes	1. Differentiate health misinformation from disinformation. 2. Understand how mistrust in the government, pharmaceutical industry, or healthcare system can contribute to vaccine decisions. 3. Role-play a patient–provider vaccine conversation.
Format	Flipped classroom
Duration	120 min

5.3.4.3 Session 4 Description

Within this 2 h session, learners analyze a blog that is authored by a physician who advises against vaccination [25]. The blog is brimming with misinformation and disinformation. The recommended format for a session on misinformation and disinformation is flipped classroom in which learners are assigned the blog as pre-reading. We recommend dividing the class into small groups where learners have the opportunity to discuss the prompts in a setting where they feel comfortable expressing their views. This can be adapted to a virtual format with several health professions and the use of Zoom breakout rooms. We developed the session for first-year pharmacy and first-year medical students. The development of clinician communication skills about vaccines is applicable to clinical pharmacists, nurses, physician assistants, and physicians, or any provider that frequently finds themselves making vaccine recommendations.

The session begins as a large group with a vignette describing a clinical encounter in which a patient has read a blog that discourages vaccination. Call on a learner to read the scenario:

> You are a third year student on rotation in the clinic. During a patient visit, your preceptor encourages the patient to get a flu shot. The patient declines the shot, saying that they recently read a study online by Dr. Kelly Brogan about flu vaccines causing depression.
>
> In private, your preceptor explains that Dr. Kelly Brogan has been mentioned a few times by patients and expresses concern that this could become problematic for the community. Your preceptor asks you to research the validity of Dr. Brogan's claims.

Immediately, learners are placed within small groups of 5–6 learners each to discuss the validity of Dr. Brogan's post related to the influenza vaccine. Learners should spend about 15–20 min in their small group before they are called back into large group discussion. Prompts should be provided to guide their discussion (Table 5.1).

Debrief as a large group by discussing the prompts. For each prompt, call on groups to summarize their group's discussion. The debrief typically takes about 15 min. Best practices are that the debrief should focus on the learners' views and cultivate a safe place for discussion.

Following the debrief, learners stay in the same small group and participate in a second activity with the goal of promoting communication skills. The second activity begins as a large group with a vignette that follows up on the previous scenario. Call on a learner to read the scenario:

> The following week, the same patient returns for a follow-up visit. Your preceptor asks you to speak to the patient about her concerns with the flu shot.

Table 5.1 Vaccine blog prompts

Analyze the hyperlinks and references within the blog.
Describe how this blog is reflective of anti-vaccination fears.
Discuss the credibility of Dr. Brogan.
Describe strategies a healthcare provider can use to explain this blog to a patient.

Table 5.2 Reflection questions

Within your interprofessional small group, what were some similarities and differences in the way each health profession approached the topic? *Focus on roles and responsibilities related to patient care.*
What are communication strategies that you would employ to enhance teamwork with other health professionals on a patient care team?
How did today's interprofessional experience change the way you will function as a member of an interprofessional team in the future?
Is there anything that you would add or change if you could repeat today's interprofessional experience?

Immediately, learners are placed back into their small groups and prompted to role-play a vaccine conversation with a patient who has read this blog. Learners take turns with one learner playing the patient and the other learner playing the clinician. To ensure that all learners have the opportunity to engage in the role-play, they should spend about 15–20 min in their small group before they are called back into large group discussion. If the session is in person, it is helpful for facilitators to walk around the room to listen to the conversations. If the session is virtual, the facilitators should rotate through breakout rooms. Debrief is a large group discussion and can include a reflection on effective vaccine metaphors (described in Sect. 5.3.2).

5.3.4.4 Session 4 Evaluation

Post session, all students complete a short-answer reflection with prompts that address effective communication skills and the roles and responsibilities of each profession in advising vaccination (Table 5.2).

5.3.5 Session 5: Empathy in Vaccine Conversations

5.3.5.1 Session 5 Rationale

Recently, the usefulness of empathetic communication in vaccine conversations with patients has gained traction [26, 27]. This communication style has gained in popularity due to the fact that previous communication styles conformed to fact-based methods that are not well received by patients [28]. During the COVID-19 pandemic, several articles showed the usefulness of an empathetic approach and provided tools for clinician use [26–28]. Given the rise of empathy education in clinical settings and these recently published papers, providing learners with a context and framework from which to draw in controversial patient interactions is important.

5.3.5.2 Session 5 Overview

Learning Outcomes	1. Understand the importance of empathy. 2. List attributes of empathy. 3. Compare and contrast empathy and sympathy. 4. Apply the use of empathy to controversial conversations.
Format	Group learning
Duration	90 min

5.3.5.3 Session 5 Description

During this 90-min session, learners observe the use of empathy, discuss empathetic communication tools, and practice using empathy with a mock vaccine-hesitant patient. There is no pre-reading or assignment to be completed prior to the session. However, learners are placed into teams of 4–5 for the three activities.

During the first activity, learners watch a short video that depicts an interaction between two people. The video begins with the couple communicating without the use of empathy. The two do not seem to listen or hear one another. However, when empathetic communication is used, there is a noticeable shift in the interaction, with clear respect and understanding. After the conclusion of the video, learners are prompted to think individually about a time when they did not feel heard or respected and how it made them feel. After a few minutes, learner teams are prompted to discuss the interaction, how well the two people communicated, and when and why the communication shifted. During debrief, facilitators interweave the attributes of empathy [29] and tools for empathetic communication [30] with the learner team responses.

The second activity centers around the use of two parallel written scenarios. The scenarios describe a situation between two of the learners' friends involved in a romantic relationship. Learners are provided one partner's side of the story in which their significant other moved to be with them while they are in school. The significant other is upset that the friend is not spending enough time with them and has started tracking their whereabouts. Learner teams are prompted to discuss how to empathize with their friend, what communication tools would they use, and what statements of empathy might they make. Then, learners are provided with the significant other's side of the story in which they feel ignored and overlooked. Learner teams are then asked how to empathize with the significant other, what communication tools would they use, and what statements of empathy might they make.

During debrief, facilitators ask learner teams to share their responses. In our experience, while learners often have an ease of understanding of the empathetic tools used in the first activity, with a more life-applicable and emotionally charged scenario, they often revert to speaking from their feelings and judgments. It is important for facilitators to discuss how empathy should be devoid of judgment, should reflect the other's emotions, and should not draw on one's own anger or pity. Rather than simply stating "I understand how you feel, I think you should do ..." learners should be prompted to make statements that reflect the other's feelings and lived experiences, ask open-ended questions, and not necessarily provide solutions or fixes to the other's problem.

The third activity applies the attributes of empathy and tools for empathetic communication to a clinical scenario involving an annual visit with a vaccine-hesitant patient. Learners are provided with the patient's medical history and then shown a short video of the patient describing her reasons for feeling hesitant about receiving a vaccine booster. The patient describes how her social community and family did not trust the medical community and how social media provided powerful anti-vaccine messages. Subsequently, learner teams are provided an empathy tool [28] to aid in gathering an understanding of the influences in the patient's life and then prompted to describe and practice their empathetic approach to a conversation about vaccination with this patient.

5.3.5.4 Session 5 Evaluation

Learners can complete a self- and peer-assessment of engagement, collaboration, and communication skills. In addition, learners can be asked to complete a post-session reflection on their confidence in applying what they learned to clinical settings. Finally, using Poll Everywhere or other live polling software, reflective prompts can be answered individually or by the team immediately following each activity. We have found this type of formative assessment helpful, particularly for the third activity, to ascertain learner perceptions of confidence in their foundational knowledge of empathy and skills to use empathy in controversial situations.

5.3.6 Session 6: Motivational Interviewing to Address Vaccine Hesitancy and Health Misinformation

5.3.6.1 Session 6 Rationale

Motivational interviewing (MI) is a valuable approach that can be used by health professionals to address vaccine hesitancy and health misinformation [31]. MI helps patients make behavioral changes to achieve a personal goal. When MI is delivered effectively, it can enhance the intrinsic motivation of patients and help them resolve hesitancy toward change.

5.3.6.2 Session 6 Overview

Learning outcomes	1. Demonstrate a relationship-centered approach to sharing information with patients. 2. Apply motivational interviewing techniques using effective communication with patients who have an expressed desire to change behavior. 3. Analyze how one's own biases and preferences impact the patient–provider relationship and health outcomes. 4. Describe clinician behaviors that positively and negatively impact a patient's willingness to share and receive information.
Format	Case-based learning and role-play
Duration	120 min

5.3.6.3 Session 6 Description

Within this 2 h session, learners implement motivational interviewing (MI) techniques to address vaccine hesitancy and highlight sources of health misinformation that are contributing to hesitancy. MI within the patient–provider conversation can facilitate change behavior with respect to vaccination. The session is most effective if the learners have already been introduced to MI earlier in the curriculum. The recommended format for a session on MI to address vaccine hesitancy is a flipped classroom in which a review of the four MI processes (engaging, focusing, evoking, and planning) is included in the pre-reading [32]. An active learning MI session is ideal for any health professional with a patient-facing role. The suggested format for this session is a case-based, small group that is facilitated by a clinician familiar with motivational interviewing. The session case scenario involves a patient in need of a recommended vaccination. Our cases involve a patient who is concerned about vaccine misinformation that they have read online. The small-group format allows learners an opportunity to implement motivational interviewing skills in a safe space. After the first hour of working through the cases, learners should use MI techniques and take turns role-playing either the patient or the clinician.

5.3.6.4 Session 6 Evaluation

Following the role-play, learners can complete a peer- and self-assessment of their implementation of core MI skills [32]. A good formative assessment is a tracking sheet that allows learners to assess their use of open-ended questions, affirmations, reflections, and summaries (OARS). Additionally, facilitators can assess students using the motivational interviewing competency assessment evaluation tool [33].

5.3.7 Session 7: Telehealth to Address Vaccine Hesitancy

5.3.7.1 Session 7 Rationale

Telehealth expands access to healthcare services, especially in rural or underserved areas. Thus, telehealth to address vaccine hesitancy is a valuable way to deliver primary care to hard-to-reach populations, improving healthcare access and equity.

5.3.7.2 Session 7 Overview

Learning outcomes	1. Utilize evidence-based communication strategies that facilitate rapport and engender trust with patients during video visits. 2. Identify factors that impact patients' readiness for vaccination. 3. Discuss barriers to vaccination with patients. 4. Recognize and respond to misinformation about vaccines. 5. Work with a patient to create a plan for getting vaccinated.
Format	Virtual patients via a telehealth visit
Duration	120 min

5.3.7.3 Session 7 Description

Within this 2 h session, learners will leverage telehealth to engage in the vaccine conversation with virtual patients. A session on telehealth works well as an interprofessional education session because telehealth often involves collaboration among healthcare providers. Ideally, the session works best in a virtual setting with simulated patients to replicate the technology utilized during a telehealth visit.

5.3.7.4 Session 7 Evaluation

Following the mock session, learners should participate in a prompted debrief to reflect on their role in the telehealth simulation and the utility of telehealth for vaccine recommendations. As a formative assessment, learners can complete a standardized peer- and self-assessment of telehealth skills [34].

5.3.8 Session 8: Simulation to Build Trust in Vaccination

5.3.8.1 Session 8 Rationale

Simulation in health professions education is a method of experiential learning and is roughly defined as a representative or artificial experience that mimics a real-life scenario [35]. Ideally, simulations will be high-fidelity virtual or in-person with standardized patients. While simulations are contrived experiences, studies have shown that simulation increases student confidence, satisfaction, knowledge acquisition, and communication skills, among others [36, 37]. This is especially true for vaccine hesitancy education. Simulations can provide powerful, nonthreatening environments wherein learners can practice their communication skills and trust building without the fear of embarrassment from other learners [37, 38].

5.3.8.2 Session 8 Overview

Learning outcomes	1. Formulate responses to concerns commonly identified by vaccine-hesitant patients and families. 2. Apply evidence-based communication techniques in simulated patient conversations. 3. Analyze the role of trust between HP and patients and the effect of mistrust on healthcare outcomes.
Format	In-person or virtual simulation
Duration	120 min

5.3.8.3 Session 8 Description

This session serves as a capstone experience that integrates previously learned concepts from the vaccine curriculum. Learner roles include gathering a history of vaccination, motivational interviewing, and administration of vaccines. An optional in-person experience can include the administration of vaccines into wearable injection pads to standardized patients. To prompt motivational interviewing, simulation scenarios should reflect a spectrum of vaccine hesitancy. For instance, one scenario can include a patient who is a partial acceptor and does not accept all needed vaccinations in the scenario. Depending on the resources available, patients can be portrayed by standardized patients, a caregiver avatar, peer learners, or video recordings.

5.3.8.4 Session 8 Evaluation

Assessment of a learner's performance in simulations can be assessed formatively or summatively. Tools to evaluate performance are available in the education literature [36]. The inclusion of a self- and peer-assessment of communication skills during the vaccine conversation helps learners to reflect on their growth in this capstone assessment. Additionally, a post-session evaluation of learner confidence and perceptions is important in capturing feedback for future sessions [17].

5.4 Conclusion

The multifaceted nature of vaccine hesitancy can make vaccine discussions with patients complex and highly charged. To address the high-stakes implications of vaccination decisions, curricular interventions and educational efforts should begin early in health professions education and continue into the clinical or applied sciences educational stages. Additionally, vaccine-specific learning experiences should cultivate communication skills and knowledge about vaccination.

Here, we have detailed eight session plans that are applicable to any health professions program, can be implemented early, and are meant to longitudinally span the entire health professions curriculum. These eight sessions incorporate active learning methodologies, including small-group clinical reasoning, case-based learning, role-play, standardized patients, telehealth, and virtual simulation experiences. Session design that integrates opportunities for deliberate practice of communication skills and flipped classroom approaches with pre-assigned work should be prioritized to promote the application of communication strategies to challenge health misinformation, build trust, and improve patient outcomes.

References

1. World Health Organization. Ten threats to global health in 2019. Available from: https://www.who.int/news-room/spotlight/ten-threats-to-global-health-in-2019.
2. Nowak GJ, Cacciatore MA. State of Vaccine Hesitancy in the United States. Pediatr Clin N Am. 2023;70(2):197–210. Available from: https://doi.org/10.1016/j.pcl.2022.11.001.
3. Maureen A, Cole J, Dodds K, Atcero M, Bada JK, Petrikova I, Worodria W. Addressing vaccine concerns through the spectrum of vaccine acceptance. Soc Sci Med. 2023;333:116146. Available from: https://doi.org/10.1016/j.socscimed.2023.116146.
4. Lip A, Pateman M, Fullerton MM, Chen HM, Bailey L, Houle S, Davidson S, Constantinescu C. Vaccine hesitancy educational tools for healthcare providers and trainees: a scoping review. Vaccine. 2023;41(1):23–35. Available from: https://doi.org/10.1016/j.vaccine.2022.09.093.
5. Kernéis S, Jacquet C, Bannay A, et al. Vaccine education of medical students: a nationwide cross-sectional survey. Am J Prev Med. 2017;53(3):e97–e104. Available from: https://doi.org/10.1016/j.amepre.2017.01.014.
6. Brauer DG, Ferguson KJ. The integrated curriculum in medical education: AMEE Guide No. 96. Med Teach. 2015;37(4):312–22. Available from: https://doi.org/10.3109/0142159x.2014.970998.
7. Woods NN. Science is fundamental: the role of biomedical knowledge in clinical reasoning. Med Educ. 2007;41(12):1173–7. Available from: https://doi.org/10.1111/j.1365-2923.2007.02911.x.
8. Schmidt HG, Machiels-Bongaerts M, Hermans H, ten Cate TJ, Venekamp R, Boshuizen HPA. The development of diagnostic competence: comparison of a problem-based, an integrated, and a conventional medical curriculum. Acad Med. 1996;71(6):658–64. Available from: https://doi.org/10.1097/00001888-199606000-00021.
9. Chase AJ, Demory ML. Counteracting vaccine misinformation: an active learning module. Med Sci Educ. 2023;33(3):1–4. Available from: https://doi.org/10.1007/s40670-023-01785-0.
10. Chase AJ, Clark MA, Rogalska A, Musselman M. Cultivating patient-physician communication about vaccination through vaccine metaphors. Med Sci Educ. 2020;30(3):1015–7. Available from: https://doi.org/10.1007/s40670-020-00981-6.
11. Thomas PA, Kern DE, Hughes MT, Chen BY. Curriculum development for medical education: a six-step approach. 3rd ed. Baltimore, MD: The Johns Hopkins University Press; 2015.
12. Tripathi T. Advances in vaccines: revolutionizing disease prevention. Sci Rep. 2023;13(1):11748. Available from: https://doi.org/10.1038/s41598-023-38798-z.
13. Center for Disease Control and Prevention. Fast facts on global immunization. Available from: https://www.cdc.gov/globalhealth/immunization/data/fast-facts.html.
14. Jackman SH, Nair D. Immunization TBL exercise. MedEdPORTAL. 2012;8:9230. Available from: https://doi.org/10.15766/mep_2374-8265.9230.
15. Lehane E, Leahy-Warren P, O'Riordan C, Savage E, Drennan J, O'Tuathaigh C, et al. Evidence-based practice education for healthcare professions: an expert view. BMJ Evid Based Med. 2018;24:103. Available from: https://doi.org/10.1136/bmjebm-2018-111019.
16. Wakefield AJ, Murch SH, Anthony A, Linnell J, Casson DM, Malik M, et al. RETRACTED: ileal-lymphoid-nodular hyperplasia, non-specific colitis, and pervasive developmental disorder in children. Lancet. 1998;351(9103):637–41. Available from: https://doi.org/10.1016/S0140-6736(97)11096-0.
17. Wiggins BL, Eddy SL, Wener-Fligner L, Freisem K, Grunspan DZ, Theobald EJ, et al. ASPECT: a survey to assess student perspective of engagement in an active-learning classroom. CBE Life Sci Educ. 2017;16(2):ar32. Available from: https://doi.org/10.1187/cbe.16-08-0244.
18. Leonardelli M, Mele F, Marrone M, Germinario CA, Tafuri S, Moscara L, et al. The effects of the COVID-19 pandemic on vaccination hesitancy: a viewpoint. Vaccines. 2023;11(7):1191. Available from: https://doi.org/10.3390/vaccines11071191.
19. U.S. Department of Health and Human Services. Immunization. Available from: https://www.hhs.gov/immunization/basics/types/index.html.

20. Centers for Disease Control and Prevention. Vaccine excipient summary. Available from: https://www.cdc.gov/vaccines/pubs/pinkbook/downloads/appendices/b/excipient-table-2.pdf.
21. Borgsteede SD, Geersing TH, Tempels-Pavlica Ž. Other excipients than PEG might cause serious hypersensitivity reactions in COVID-19 vaccines. Allergy. 2021;76(6):1941. Available from: https://doi.org/10.1111/all.14774.
22. Centers for Disease Control and Prevention. Thimerosal and Vaccines. Available from: https://www.cdc.gov/vaccinesafety/concerns/thimerosal/index.html.
23. Caballero ML, Krantz MS, Quirce S, Phillips EJ, Stone CA Jr. Hidden dangers: recognizing excipients as potential causes of drug and vaccine hypersensitivity reactions. J Allergy Clin Immunol Pract. 2021;9(8):2968–82. Available from: https://doi.org/10.1016/j.jaip.2021.03.002.
24. Do Nascimento IJB, Pizarro AB, Almeida JM, Azzopardi-Muscat N, Gonçalves MA, Björklund M, Novillo-Ortiz D. Infodemics and health misinformation: a systematic review of reviews. Bull World Health Organ. 2022;100(9):544. Available from: https://doi.org/10.2471/BLT.21.287654.
25. Kelly Brogan MD. Could the flu shot make you depressed? Available from: https://www.kellybroganmd.com/blog/could-the-flu-shot-make-you-depressed.
26. Poland CM, Ratishvili T. Vaccine hesitancy and health care providers: using the preferred cognitive styles and decision-making model and empathy tool to make progress. Vaccine: X. 2022;11:100174. Available from: https://doi.org/10.1016/j.jvacx.2022.100174.
27. Holford D, Schmid P, Fasce A, Lewandowsky S. The empathetic refutational interview to tackle vaccine misconceptions: four randomized experiments. Health Psychol. 2024;43:426. Available from: https://doi.org/10.1037/hea0001354.
28. Poland CM, Matthews AK, Poland GA. Improving COVID-19 vaccine acceptance: including insights from human decision-making under conditions of uncertainty and human-centered design. Vaccine. 2021;39(11):1547–50. Available from: https://doi.org/10.1016/j.vaccine.2021.02.008.
29. Wiseman T. A concept analysis of empathy. J Adv Nurs. 1996;23(6):1162–7. Available from: https://10.1046/j.1365-2648.1996.12213.x.
30. Stubbe DE. Engaging the "Difficult" patient: strengthening empathic communication skills. Focus. 2022;20(4):413–5. Available from: https://doi.org/10.1176/appi.focus.20220067.
31. Jamison KC, Ahmed AH, Spoerner DA, Kinney D. Best shot: a motivational interviewing approach to address vaccine hesitancy in pediatric outpatient settings. J Pediatr Nurs. 2022;67:124–31. https://doi.org/10.1016/j.pedn.2022.08.012.
32. Miller WR, Rollnick S. Motivational interviewing: Helping people change. 3rd ed. New York: Guilford Press; 2013.
33. Vossen J, Burduli E, Barbosa-Leiker C. Reliability and validity testing. Washington State University; 2018. Motivational Interviewing Competency Assessment (MICA). Available at: www.micacoding.com.
34. Schroeder MN, Lengel AJ. Evaluation of a rubric to assess pharmacy student performance in a telehealth simulation exercise. Am J Pharm Educ. 2022;86(8):ajpe8778. https://doi.org/10.5688/ajpe8778.
35. Al-Elq AH. Simulation-based medical teaching and learning. J Fam Community Med. 2010;17(1):35–40. Available from: https://doi.org/10.4103/1319-1683.68787.
36. Hekel BE, Dugger J, Pullis BR, Cron S, Edwards AP. Vaccine hesitancy: developing competency in nursing students through simulation. Nurse Educ. 2024;49(2):E62–7. Available from: https://doi.org/10.1097/NNE.0000000000001505.
37. Real FJ, DeBlasio D, Beck AF, Ollberding NJ, Davis D, Cruse B, et al. A virtual reality curriculum for pediatric residents decreases rates of influenza vaccine refusal. Acad Pediatr. 2017;17(4):431–5. Available from: https://doi.org/10.1016/j.acap.2017.01.010.
38. Norton ZS, Olson KB, Sanguino SM. Addressing vaccine hesitancy through a comprehensive resident vaccine curriculum. MedEdPORTAL. 2022;18:11292. Available from: https://doi.org/10.15766/mep_2374-8265.11292.

Chapter 6
Interprofessional Instructional Design Strategies to Mitigate Vaccine Misinformation, Disinformation, and Mistrust

William A. Prescott, Jr., Kelly Foltz-Ramos, Jessica S. Kruger, Ijeoma S. Anadi, and Nicholas M. Fusco

6.1 Introduction

The explosion of medical misinformation and disinformation on social media is a growing global public health concern [60]. In the case of misinformation, there is a communication of fallacies that may or may not be intentional. Disinformation, in contrast, entails an intentional dissemination of false information with the intent to mislead [19]. Both are perpetuated by complex, interdependent social and political factors and affect the ability of health workers to provide high-quality care and for patients to make decisions about their health based on credible information. Vaccine hesitancy exemplifies how myths and misperceptions driven by mis- and disinformation can affect direct patient care and population health [24, 25, 42, 53, 86].

W. A. Prescott, Jr. (✉) · I. S. Anadi · N. M. Fusco
Department of Pharmacy Practice, University at Buffalo School of Pharmacy and Pharmaceutical Sciences, Buffalo, NY, USA
e-mail: prescott@buffalo.edu; ijeomaan@buffalo.edu; nmfusco@buffalo.edu

K. Foltz-Ramos
Department of Simulation and Innovation, University at Buffalo School of Nursing, Buffalo, NY, USA
e-mail: foltz@buffalo.edu

J. S. Kruger
Department of Community Health and Health Behavior, University at Buffalo School of Public Health and Health Professions, Buffalo, NY, USA
e-mail: jskruger@buffalo.edu

A. J. Chase et al. (eds.), *Vaccine Hesitancy Curriculum*,
https://doi.org/10.1007/978-3-031-88668-3_6

Vaccine hesitancy is a delay in acceptance or refusal to vaccinate, despite the availability of vaccines [63]. Identified as a top-10 threat to global health by the World Health Organization in 2019 [104], vaccine hesitancy is influenced by confidence, complacency, and convenience [63]. Those who spread mis- and disinformation about vaccines focus on the first two aspects, targeting the confidence patients have in the safety and effectiveness of vaccines and downplaying the need for and importance of vaccination. Conversations about vaccine hesitancy are challenging; however, because vaccine hesitancy exists on a continuum between total acceptance and complete refusal, with vaccine-hesitant patients residing in the middle [63], conversing with patients about their concerns is imperative if a health worker is to influence change. A successful outcome necessitates health workers have a good working knowledge of vaccines, strong interpersonal skills, and that they be aware of the concerns patients may have.

Health workers can, and often do, unilaterally address patient (and caregiver) concerns relating to vaccination. However, an interprofessional, team-based approach to mitigating vaccine hesitancy may be as effective, if not more so. Furthermore, such an approach may lighten the workload on any one health worker [77]. Interprofessional education (IPE) provides an opportunity to teach students the value of interprofessional collaborative practice (IPCP), the implications mis- and disinformation can have on patient care and public health, and how to best approach conversations about vaccine hesitancy. This chapter will discuss interprofessional instructional design strategies that can be used in higher education to equip health occupations students with the knowledge and skills they need to mitigate vaccine misinformation, disinformation, and mistrust.

6.2 Addressing the Pervasive Issue of Medical Misinformation and Disinformation

Misinformation and disinformation existed long before the Information Age. This is highlighted by vaccine hesitancy, an issue that has been a public health concern ever since the widespread use of the first vaccine for smallpox in the 1800s [39]. The advent of the internet and social media provided means for rapid, widespread dissemination of content, including both scientifically sound and inaccurate information about vaccines [54, 79]. This presents a challenge for patients seeking health information as it may seem that there exists no consensus on a given topic or worse, that validated sources of information are not credible. This can bring about confusion and mistrust, prompting some individuals to disengage from health information seeking, avoid health care, or make decisions detrimental to their health and the health of those within their sphere of influence [14]. A perfect example is how disinformation about the measles/mumps/rubella (MMR) vaccine in the late 1900s and early 2000s prompted widespread mis- and disinformation that negatively impacted confidence in the safety of the MMR vaccine [39]. The myths surrounding the risks of MMR vaccination, most importantly an association with autism, were founded on falsified research from a discredited physician-researcher; despite a plethora of data disproving a causal relationship, patient concerns about the safety of the MMR vaccine persist [1].

The design of social media and the algorithms they employ have exacerbated the spread of mis- and disinformation, an issue that garnered attention during the Coronavirus Disease 19 (COVID-19) pandemic when public health measures, including vaccination, were polarizing issues driven by unfounded stories, conspiracy theories, and pseudoscience. In the case of Facebook and X (formally Twitter), a person's feed is tailored to their preferences or beliefs, which contributes to what is known as the "echo chamber effect," where repetitive exposure to content leads to confirmation bias, increasing the believability and shareability of content [13]. A patient may neglect opposing perspectives and viewpoints that conflict with their own [14], and the longer their beliefs persist without challenge, the more likely it is to influence health behaviors, a phenomenon termed the "illusory truth effect" [5]. In this scenario, a patient may propagate mis- and disinformation, possibly unknowingly and without malice, extending the reach of uncredible sources. It is unclear how the recent introduction of artificial intelligence (AI) will affect the prevalence of mis- and disinformation. While it may be utilized to generate and disseminate credible information, it can just as easily be manipulated to promulgate mis- and disinformation. Therefore, it is vital that both patients and the healthcare community be skilled in critically evaluating online content, including information generated by AI.

Key stakeholders positioned to mitigate the negative impact of health mis- and disinformation include health workers, educators, and the public. Patients will seek out health information; efforts that improve their skills in separating good and bad advice can have a profound impact on individual and public health efforts. It has been established that patients place a high-level trust in health workers [26, 34], and while they may seek information from multiple sources, most do rely on their health provider to guide decisions that are important to their health and wellbeing [95]. While health workers serve as a source of credible medical information, educators are uniquely positioned to improve the public's digital literacy and basic understanding of vaccines. The Office of the Surgeon General has advised that media, digital, data, science, and health literacy programs be implemented across primary (elementary), secondary, post-secondary, and community settings [69]. Lastly, academicians can work to quantify the harm of health mis- and disinformation, conceive and evaluate strategies for combatting it, and advocate for policies that address mis- and disinformation in healthcare.

6.3 Interprofessional Instructional Design Strategies to Mitigate Misinformation and Disinformation

6.3.1 Applying Educational Theory to Design Learning

Applying educational theory to the design of IPE learning experiences that teach health occupations students about mis/disinformation and vaccine hesitancy encourages the use of effective, evidence-based pedagogy. When sound pedagogies are employed, both learning and retention are enhanced, equipping students with the skills they need to mitigate these critical public health challenges [37]. Educational theories that should be utilized include cognitive load theory, experiential learning theory, and the theory of deliberate practice.

Cognitive Load Theory pertains to how an individual's cognitive resources are allocated during the learning process [72, 91]. This theory can be used to optimize the design of IPE programs that involve health workers from various disciplines [43]. The three types of cognitive load are intrinsic, extraneous, and germane [72, 73]. Intrinsic Cognitive Load refers to the inherent complexity of the learning tasks. In IPE, it can involve a working memory of the roles and responsibilities of different health professions, understanding the topic, and appreciating how to effectively communicate and collaborate. Extraneous Cognitive Load is related to the instructional design and environment. In IPE, this can be amplified by the provision of confusing or poorly structured materials, unclear instructions, or a lack of coordination in team activities. Germane Cognitive Load is the cognitive effort dedicated to learning and understanding. In IPE, it includes activities that promote teamwork, communication, and the acquisition of knowledge about the focus and value of other health professions.

Applying cognitive load theory to IPE involves designing learning activities and materials in a way that minimizes extraneous cognitive load, effectively manages intrinsic cognitive load, and maximizes germane cognitive load. To minimize extraneous load, educators should ensure that instructional materials are well-organized, instructions are clear, and that the learning environment supports effective teamwork. To manage intrinsic load, educators can design pre-session educational materials intended to prepare students for the scenario, revisiting previously learned content and breaking down complex concepts into manageable units. To enhance germane load, educators need to provide opportunities for learners to actively engage with content and discuss interprofessional issues, provide feedback to help students learn from their mistakes, and engage students in reflective debriefing sessions [83]. For instance, educators might offer pre-session educational modules or virtual simulations intended to prepare students for the IPE activity, paired with well-designed and validated case-based simulations, role-playing exercises, and team projects to facilitate interprofessional learning [59]. When done correctly, applying this theory to IPE helps learners focus on understanding and applying interprofessional collaboration concepts and skills without being overwhelmed by intrinsic and extrinsic cognitive demands [43].

Experiential Learning Theory, also known as Kolb's Theory of Experiential Learning, emphasizes the importance of learning through direct experience and active engagement [48, 55]. In the context of IPE, it provides a framework for health workers from different disciplines to learn and collaborate effectively by engaging in real-world experiences, reflection, and problem-solving [21]. IPE based on experiential learning theory promotes a holistic approach to health professions education, where students from various disciplines actively engage with one another in simulated or actual clinical environments [16, 75]. This approach helps learners acquire knowledge and develop the skills and attitudes necessary for effective collaboration and patient-centered care, improving patient outcomes and the quality of healthcare services [16].

Experiential learning theory emphasizes the idea that learning is most effective when it is based on personal experience and reflection [48, 55]. It is often represented as a four-stage learning cycle: First, concrete experience, where the learner encounters a new experience or situation; second, reflective observation, where the learner reflects on that experience; third, abstract conceptualization, where the learner attempts to make sense of the experience by developing abstract concepts or theories; and fourth, active experimentation, where the learner applies the new knowledge or theories to real-world situations. The result is one where students take what they have learned and put it into practice, testing their ideas, trying out new strategies, and gaining additional experience. This theory has been successfully applied in health professions education [71]. Table 6.1 describes how the principles of experiential learning theory can be applied to IPE, so it is of benefit to health occupations students.

The Theory of Deliberate Practice highlights the role of focused and intentional practice in developing expertise in a particular field [20]. This theory is well suited for IPE as it underscores the importance of intentional and structured learning experiences that focus on improving collaboration and teamwork. In the context of IPE, this can entail repeated opportunities to practice teamwork and collaboration through simulation and real-world patient care experiences [93]. Following each IPE experience, learners should take time to reflect on the simulation/real-world experience, their strengths and weaknesses, and opportunities for improvement. Through repeated, challenging, and reflective practice, health occupations students can enhance their abilities to provide high-quality patient-centered care through IPCP [98] Table 6.2 provides an example of how deliberate practice theory can be applied to IPE.

6.3.2 Interprofessional Education Strategies

To effectively address mis- and disinformation, a health worker needs a firm grasp of subject material and current events, strong interpersonal skills, and an appreciation for how other health workers can contribute to the conversation. Foundational content pertaining to profession-specific duties should be covered within individual

Table 6.1 Application of experiential learning theory principles to interprofessional education

Stage	Activity	Description	Learning Objectives
Concrete experience	Case studies, simulations	Provide real-world experiences related to vaccine mis/disinformation and hesitancy. Students analyze and engage in scenarios involving real-life challenges and misinformation issues in vaccination.	Develop an understanding of real-world challenges related to vaccine mis/disinformation and hesitancy. Identify common misconceptions and issues contributing to vaccine mistrust. Experience the emotional and cognitive aspects associated with these challenges.
Reflective observation	Debriefing, group discussions, and journaling	Encourage students to reflect on their experiences, observations, and emotions. Students share their observations with peers through group discussions and reflective journaling. They discuss what they observed, what worked, what did not work, and how it made them feel.	Foster critical thinking about their experiences and observations. Promote the ability to articulate and communicate their insights and feelings to peers. Develop empathy and understanding of diverse perspectives regarding vaccine hesitancy and mis/disinformation.
Abstract conceptualization	Debriefing, group discussions, lectures, readings, and research	Guide learners in drawing conclusions and creating general principles. Students will engage in discussions, readings, and research to analyze their experiences, integrate existing knowledge, and seek new information to better understand the issues.	Develop a deeper understanding of the underlying factors contributing to vaccine mis/disinformation and hesitancy. Encourage the formulation of general principles and theories related to the topic. Enhance research and critical analysis skills.
Active experimentation	Clinical practice, designing interventions, role-playing	Allow students to apply their conclusions in practical settings. Students will design and test strategies and interventions to address vaccine mis/disinformation and hesitancy, engaging in role-playing scenarios to evaluate the effectiveness of their strategies.	Develop problem-solving and intervention design skills. Apply theoretical knowledge to real-world situations. Evaluate the effectiveness of their strategies and interventions. Enhance communication and teamwork skills in an interprofessional context.

Table 6.2 Application of deliberate practice theory in interprofessional education, example

Stage	Activity	Description	Learning Objectives
Scenario development	Design of vaccine misinformation scenarios	Faculty creates scenarios where interprofessional students must address vaccine mis/disinformation and mistrust. The scenarios should include realistic patient profiles with different concerns.	To expose students to vaccine mis/disinformation. To provide a realistic context for addressing mistrust.
Orientation	Simulation pre-briefing	Faculty or facilitators introduce students to the simulation platform and explain the objectives of the exercise.	To familiarize students with the purpose and process of the simulation.
Simulation	Engagement in deliberate practice	Students participate in multiple rounds of simulation, with each round presenting a different scenario or patient profile. They must work together to address vaccine mis/disinformation and mistrust.	To practice patient communication and counseling skills in an interprofessional setting, adapting strategy to various scenarios.
Feedback & reflection	Simulation debriefing	Students receive feedback from faculty or peers and engage in a reflection session centered on the experience, their performance, and opportunities for improvement. At the end, they discuss their overall progress and lessons learned in addressing vaccine misinformation and mistrust.	To encourage self-assessment and reflection. To identify strengths and areas for growth. To facilitate a comprehensive reflection on the experience.

health professions curricula, permitting the use of IPE to deepen a student's understanding and to introduce IPCP principles and broader issues facing the healthcare community.

There are a variety of techniques that can be employed in IPE to equip health occupations students to engage patients who may hold false or incorrect beliefs rooted in mis- and disinformation, including but not limited to active listening, motivational interviewing, and best practices such as using a structured, tailored approach to address vaccine-related concerns [95]. When interacting with patients, it is important the health worker understands what the patient or caregiver is saying. This involves active listening and confirming responses, which necessitates skills in nonverbal communication, showing empathy, asking the right types of questions, and reflecting on what the patient has said [95]. Furthermore, this approach can help build trusting relationships with patients, which opens the door for countering misplaced beliefs like vaccine hesitancy. Motivational interviewing, a "directive, client-centered counseling style for collaborating with clients to enact a behavior change" [65], is another approach that can be used by health workers. Unlike typical patient educational strategies, motivational interviewing is a collaborative conversation that empowers the patient to make a commitment or a change [66]. Teaching health occupations students to respond to mis- and disinformation with empathy, curiosity, and compassion using a core set of counseling skills (e.g., open-ended questions, affirmations, reflections, and summary statements), in an individualized manner, can help the student and patient arrive at a shared goal or focus for the interaction, evoke motivation for change, and if appropriate, create plans to accomplish identified goals [87]. These skills can be learned; providing time and space in the IPE curriculum to practice active listening and motivational interviewing, in both neutral and tense situations, is critical to the development of a practice-ready health occupations student.

The best approach, in our experience, to equip students with the knowledge and skills they need to mitigate vaccine mis- and disinformation and mistrust, is to introduce these skills at the individual college/school-level and grow these skills through IPE. Training students how to engage in active listening and motivational interviewing through virtual simulation and in-person simulated experiences using standardized patients provides a safe, immersive learning environment and equips them for practice. When done interprofessionally, it has an added benefit of learning from another member of the healthcare team, which provides the learner with insight as to what they and other members of the team can contribute, while also teaching the value of collaboration. For example, students need foundational knowledge in order to address vaccine hesitancy, such as the safety and effectiveness of vaccines and an understanding of the diseases they prevent. They also need to develop certain skills, such as how to navigate health information technology and communicating with patients. These aspects can be effectively covered through didactic and skills courses at the individual college/school-level and revisited through pre-session educational modules. In contrast, how to effectively interact with vaccine-hesitant patients and caregivers, and how to work as a team to dispel myths and misperceptions rooted in mis- and disinformation to encourage vaccination, are better suited for an advanced, interactive IPE setting.

6.3.3 Challenges with Interprofessional Education

Students desire to gain experience in realistic scenarios that they are likely to encounter in practice [64]. IPE is a promising approach to accomplish this because it can be immersive in design and may be used to prepare health occupations students for collaborative, patient-centered practice [105]. The overarching goal of IPE is to foster teamwork, communication, and mutual understanding among students from different healthcare disciplines [47]. The Interprofessional Education Collaborative (IPEC®) has established core competencies intended to ensure that new and current health workers are able to integrate knowledge, skills, and values/attitudes essential for patient-centered, community- and population-oriented IPCP [47]. While the benefits are evident, the process of designing and implementing effective IPE is not without challenges. There are five major challenges to IPE: (1) Institutional support, (2) Geography and infrastructure, (3) Programmatic structure, (4) Practice environment and culture, and (5) Assessment approaches.

6.3.3.1 Institutional Support

Institutional support is of utmost importance. To realize this, it is critical that health professions programs develop a shared vision for IPE and encourage their faculty to forge collaborative relationships with other health professions educators across campus. Equally important is administrator buy-in as these individuals control the allocation of faculty resources, provision of protected time (and credit for teaching) for faculty, and allocation of monetary resources to fund IPE programming. If one or more of these attributes are lacking, the quality of and engagement in IPE can be compromised [99, 102].

6.3.3.2 Geography and Infrastructure

Second, geography and infrastructure can present challenges. For example, a small college with a single health professions program will face challenges that a larger university with an academic health center will not. To offer IPE opportunities to their students, these institutions may need to establish collaborations with health professions schools that are outside their home institution. As another example, universities with multiple campuses face distance education challenges. Technology, such as online learning, can help overcome this barrier to IPE but necessitates attention to facilitator training and faculty development to ensure technology is used in a way that encourages learning [106].

6.3.3.3 Programmatic Structure

Third, programmatic structure, including scheduling, faculty/student availability, curricular demands, and profession-specific accreditation standards, is a long-standing barrier to executing an effective IPE program [101]. Given the extensive curricular demands of health professions programs, which must work within the campus' physical space confines, identifying time to deliver IPE experiences can be trying, particularly in a post-pandemic world where workforce demands have stressed the bandwidth of clinical and teaching faculty [106]. Likewise, coordinating schedules among students from different health professions programs and/or other institutions can be difficult to navigate without advanced planning and flexibility. Although one-off events may be simpler to arrange, they are less likely to yield meaningful changes in student knowledge, skills, or attitudes if not reinforced at another time [102]. Furthermore, harmonizing discipline-specific outcomes and interprofessional learning outcomes across multiple degree programs and multiple levels of learners within these programs requires extensive collaboration and planning [41].

6.3.3.4 Practice Environment and Culture

Fourth, while a university may have successfully implemented an IPE curriculum, it is equally important they and their practice site partners carry these values over to practice. If IPCP is not modeled in experiential learning environments, faculty and students alike may not find these experiences valuable and rewarding [64]. While it is possible for students to develop basic skills in communication and collaboration in the classroom, neglecting the influences of hierarchy, power imbalances, and professional identity on the practice side impedes a student's ability to apply these skills to practice [40]. University and practice site leadership play a critical role in modeling and endorsing desired interprofessional competencies, and there needs to be alignment between organizational policies, educational systems, and culture to achieve lasting solutions [84].

6.3.3.5 Assessment Approaches

Lastly, traditional assessment methods may not effectively measure the outcomes of IPE, which focus on interprofessional competencies such as teamwork and collaboration. Designing appropriate assessment tools and approaches that accurately evaluate student abilities in these areas is a persistent challenge [82]. The assessment process must align with the program's objectives and provide meaningful insight into student readiness for collaborative practice [102]. Achieving this balance often requires research, development, and validation of new assessment strategies, particularly when training a large, diverse group of learners.

Overcoming these challenges demands a coordinated effort among educators, higher education institutions, and healthcare organizations. By recognizing the above-mentioned complexities and working together to develop innovative solutions, health professions education can continue to evolve in a way that effectively prepares students to meet the demands of a dynamic and collaborative healthcare landscape. The following section provides general recommendations for planning and sustaining an effective IPE program.

6.3.4 Planning Effective Interprofessional Education Activities for Health Occupations Students

Designing and implementing an effective IPE program requires a stepwise process. A fundamental step in planning IPE is to define clear and specific learning objectives, ideally adapted from validated competency frameworks. Several validated competency frameworks exist, including the Canadian Interprofessional Health Collaborative [12] and the IPEC® Core Competencies for Interprofessional

Collaborative Practice [47]. The IPEC® competency framework has been influential in informing accreditation practices for health professions education, as evidenced by their inclusion in the national guideline published by the Health Professions Accreditors Collaborative (HPAC) and [36] the National Center for Interprofessional Practice and Education in 2019 [67]. The four competencies defined by IPEC® are (1) values and ethics, (2) roles and responsibilities, (3) communication, and (4) teams and teamwork [47]. Student acquisition of interprofessional collaborative competencies is a longitudinal process [46]. Thus, the professional development of health occupations students may be encouraged by establishing a progressive framework to guide IPE over the course of the students' academic program [96].

Pedagogical approaches and methods for assessment need to be defined and aligned with the established learning outcomes. IPE activities should be representative of the participating health-professions and should emphasize practical, real-world scenarios that mirror the complexities of practice. Interdependence in shared problem-solving is critical, as students may disengage if they determine that their professional knowledge or skills are irrelevant to an IPE activity [100]. Furthermore, the activity and its associated learning objectives should align with the level of experience of the learner. For example, it may be challenging for students to apply themselves in the context of interprofessional team dynamics if they lack or have a limited understanding of their own professional identity. Therefore, considering professional identity takes time to develop [35], an activity that requires students to understand their professional identify may be better situated later in the IPE curriculum.

Assessment is critical; however, review of IPE interventions have indicated that assessment methods vary widely [23], generally lack rigorous design [82], and often rely on some level of student self-report rather than independent observation [23]. Several assessment tools exist, and a systematic review has characterized how they can be employed based on the desired assessment framework [88]. The National Center for Interprofessional Practice and Education has compiled many resources, including assessment tools, which are helpful to educators when designing and assessing IPE [67]. While instructors may desire a rigorous IPE assessment, it is important to be mindful that IPE should be administered in a safe learning environment [64]. Furthermore, establishing a supportive and inclusive learning environment is critical to encourage participation and active engagement in IPE experiences [7–9].

An impactful IPE experience requires interaction between faculty and students. Faculty may be inclined to teach to students through information transfer; however, guiding a robust conversation is a preferred approach. While facilitating an interprofessional group of learners is, in theory, comparable to facilitating a group consisting of a single health profession, faculty may need to adjust their strategy to effectively connect with and engage students from different professions [85]. Frameworks such as train-the-trainer have been employed to scale the number of trained faculty facilitators for IPE [4]. To effectively facilitate an IPE session, health professions faculty should strive to:

- Be professionally neutral
- Recognize diversity in students' background, both professionally and culturally
- Be aware of perceived professional hierarchy and stereotypical beliefs about professions
- Realize students may lack appreciation of the roles/responsibilities of other health professions
- Value the distinctive experience and expertise of each participating student
- Pose thought-provoking questions and use active-listening and probing techniques
- Clarify professional jargon
- Encourage discussion around the fundamentals of the IPEC® Core Competencies
- Promote the benefits of IPE for teamwork and link effective team collaboration to patient care

The success of an IPE program hinges on institutional support and active participation from stakeholders, including faculty and administrators from various health professions, students, and practicing health workers. Engaging stakeholders early in the planning process is critical as their expertise, experience, insight, and support are invaluable for shaping a relevant, effective, and sustainable program. The IPEC Institutional Assessment Instrument is available and can be used to assess the capacity for high-quality programmatic IPE at an institution and to advocate for needed resources [107]. A thoughtfully designed IPE program, supported by the institution and its stakeholders, serves to prepare health occupations students for IPCP and to provide patient-centered care centered on optimizing healthcare outcomes. Planning and implementing such a program requires a strategic approach that considers the diverse needs of learners, the collaborative nature of healthcare practice, and the goals of each health professions program. By following these general tips and tailoring the program to the organization, health professions educators can design and implement valuable learning experiences that equip future health workers with the skills and mindset necessary for IPCP.

6.4 Interprofessional Instructional Design Strategies: Case Studies/Best Practices

The education of health occupations students in the IPE setting should promote active engagement in the learning process. Furthermore, pedagogy should promote interaction with other health occupations students. We recommend three approaches that accomplish both goals, simulation-based learning, team-based learning, and gamification. Approaches like this are widely favored methods for IPE because they engage students in collaborative teams and facilitate skill development, the exploration of roles, the application of diverse communication techniques, and team development [101].

6.4.1 Simulation-Based Learning

Simulation-based learning has long been used in health professions education to train students in a safe, immersive environment that mimics real-life. In this educational setting, students can, without consequence, make mistakes and learn from them. Best practices in interprofessional instructional design related to simulation revolve around creating effective learning experiences that prepare health occupations students from various disciplines to work collaboratively in real-world healthcare settings [45].

Simulation may be done virtually or in-person. Virtual desktop-based simulation in IPE offers a safe, flexible, and scalable platform for practical, evidence-based learning. It allows students to engage in complex healthcare scenarios, make decisions, receive immediate feedback, and reflect on their experiences [62]. In a risk-free setting, they can learn from mistakes, adapt, and develop/refine their trade [94]. This approach not only exposes learners to the perspectives of different healthcare disciplines but also prepares them for effective teamwork. Virtual simulation is often used to prepare students for in-person simulation [32, 33, 62, 94]. In-person simulation in IPE offers additional benefits, namely realism through direct interaction with high-fidelity human patient simulators [29] or face-to-face encounters with living, breathing human beings [32, 33].

The first element to consider when designing a simulation is setting clear learning objectives with a focus on teamwork development, communication, and clinical skills. Furthermore, scenarios should be realistic, reflecting the complexities and challenges of interprofessional collaboration in healthcare. The integration of standardized patients into simulations, when best practices are followed, adds realism and value to the IPE experience [45]. Standardized participants should be well-trained to authentically portray patients, family members, or other health workers, which, if done correctly, enhances the realism of the simulation. Also, if desired and appropriately trained, standardized patients can evaluate student performance, allowing faculty to focus on the debriefing [2].

The second essential component is a structured, post-simulation debriefing and reflection with all participating health occupations students. This debriefing, which is led by trained faculty facilitators, allows participants to discuss their simulated experience, reflect on their performance, and provide feedback to one another [57, 74]. Considering performance feedback is not a duty of the facilitator, the provision of peer feedback can help students identify areas where they are strong and areas in which they can improve. Alternatively, incorporating feedback mechanisms such as video recording or real-time, generalized feedback from instructors not engaged in facilitation helps participants gauge their performance and practice-readiness, facilitating growth and skill development.

Lastly, a collaborative learning environment is critical in interprofessional instructional design. Creating physical and virtual spaces that promote teamwork and communication is essential. Pre-briefing sessions should be conducted to prepare participants for the simulation and to set expectations; this can reduce anxiety and ensure that everyone understands their roles [58]. A culture of continuous improvement is encouraged, allowing for iterative design based on participant feedback and observed outcomes [32, 33]. By following these best practices, educators can create impactful interprofessional simulations that prepare health workers to excel in interdisciplinary healthcare environments, enhancing their readiness for IPCP.

6.4.2 Team-Based Learning

Team-based learning, originally developed in the 1970s, has been widely used in health professions education, including dentistry, medicine, nursing, pharmacy, and physical therapy [7, 8, 10, 17, 49, 51, 61, 68, 70, 76, 89]. This way of teaching, often an aspect of the flipped classroom format, is organized into three phases. First, the "preparatory" phase directs students to engage with pre-class learning materials on their own and at their own pace, to establish a foundational understanding of the topic. Second, the "readiness assurance" phase requires students to complete an in-class individual assessment, which holds them accountable for the pre-class work, followed by a group assessment, which facilitates peer-to-peer teaching. The "application phase," which typically entails case-based learning or simulation, is intended to promote higher-level learning. Team-based learning can prepare health occupations students for real-world healthcare scenarios [10, 51] and has demonstrated utility in IPE [6]. This active learning approach helps students shape their professional identity by enhancing self-awareness and facilitating deeper insight into their own profession and that of peers within other healthcare disciplines [3, 6–8]. Furthermore, team-based learning can enhance communication skills and promote collaboration, essential skills of a health worker [51, 56, 76, 89]. The skills developed through team-based learning in IPE can help prepare health occupations students to engage in IPCP to cultivate safe, effective healthcare. A newer approach that encourages team-based learning is gamification, as will be discussed in the next section.

6.4.3 Gamification

Gamification, an emerging and innovative approach in IPE that harnesses the principles of game design to engage students in collaborative learning experiences, has gained traction in health professions education [97]. This educational approach engages and motivates learners by allowing them to practice critical thinking, decision-making, and communication skills while addressing real-world challenges [15]. It encompasses various elements, including video games and escape rooms, to promote teamwork, communication, and problem-solving skills among interdisciplinary teams [22, 27, 28, 30, 31, 33, 38, 44, 50]. These serious games designed for

IPE often simulate complex healthcare scenarios, challenging learners to work together to diagnose, treat, and make informed patient care decisions [103]. The use of escape rooms is a good example of serious gaming. This interactive activity, which entails uncovering clues, solving puzzles, and accomplishing tasks to successfully "escape the room" within a specific timeframe, necessitates health occupations students approach health-related problems using critical thinking and teamwork, skills that are vital for effective IPCP [22, 27, 28, 31, 33, 38, 44].

Studies examining academic outcomes and student perceptions of serious games in IPE reveal higher scores on knowledge assessments and increased interprofessional socialization and self-confidence among students [22, 30–33, 44]. Through gamification, students gain a deeper understanding of various health professions and express enjoyment and engagement as they recognize how they can depend on the expertise of other colleagues for specific aspects of patient care in the future [30–33, 38]. A 2021 review published by van Gaalen and colleagues suggests potential benefits to student learning outcomes in health professions education, especially when employing game attributes intended to improve learning behaviors and attitudes toward learning [97].

Serious games offer an interactive and immersive learning environment, allowing participants to gain practical experience and apply their knowledge in a risk-free setting. By gamifying the learning process, participants become more motivated and invested in their educational activities. When paired with IPE, gamification is a powerful means for instilling teamwork and problem-solving skills in students.

6.5 Future Directions

6.5.1 Emerging Technologies

Emerging technologies are poised to significantly impact interprofessional instructional design strategies aimed at mitigating vaccine misinformation and mistrust. Most notably, virtual reality (VR) and augmented reality (AR) can create highly immersive and realistic training environments where students from various healthcare disciplines collaborate to address vaccine-related challenges [90]. Simulations using VR and AR are revolutionizing IPE within the healthcare field.

VR simulation provides a highly immersive and realistic environment for health workers to collaborate and refine their skills in a safe and controlled manner. This approach has the potential to transcend geographical boundaries, creating opportunities for a more diverse community of learners. It is also cost-effective and scalable, making it a valuable resource to invest in for the healthcare academic setting [52]. VR simulation can be used to teach soft skills like teamwork and communication, as well as clinical decision-making and direct patient care [80, 81]. As technology continues to advance, VR simulation is poised to become an integral part of IPE.

In contrast to VR, AR simulation blends digital information with the real world, allowing health workers to practice their clinical skills, teamwork, and communication in authentic clinical settings [11]. These dynamic and adaptable learning experiences are accessible to a broader audience because they eliminate the need for physical proximity. Learners can utilize wearable AR devices to access real-time information and support, which enhances their clinical expertise. The future of IPE is expected to be shaped by AR simulation, which empowers health workers to apply their knowledge directly in actual clinical contexts [18].

6.5.2 K-12 Education

By teaching grade-school students about bacteria and viruses, vaccines, and how our immune system works, K-12 education can play a key role in confronting mis/disinformation and mistrust in vaccines [78]. Educational resources to support K-12 science curricula, tailored to the level of learner, are freely available through the Vaccine Education Center at the Children's Hospital of Philadelphia (https://vaccinemakers.org/). One unit, designed for high school students, is dedicated to disease and vaccination.

The immediate benefit of educating primary and secondary students about vaccines and navigating online resources is first, to help them understand what vaccines are and why they need them, and second, to help them forge direct connections between science and their daily lives. The current cohort of elementary, middle-, and high-school students lived through the global COVID-19 pandemic, an event that impacted their schooling and life in general. The pandemic serves as a timely example that depicts how vaccination can help society return to normalcy. Furthermore, it directly connects with the life-experience of these children and adolescents, in a way that is not too dissimilar to what their grandparents experienced with poliomyelitis during the 1940s and 1950s. In addition to these immediate benefits, there may also be a longer-term impact of teaching this topic in K-12 education, namely helping students understand vaccine basics and how to distinguish between valid and misinformation. The Disease and Vaccination unit offered through the Vaccine Makers Project includes a lesson intended to teach students the difference between accurate and inaccurate information and examine the ways that information spreads via social media networks, skills that can be applied beyond vaccines [92].

Educating K-12 students on vaccines and mis/disinformation serves to equip the next generation with the knowledge and skills they need to make informed decisions as adults, not only for themselves but also for their children. Institutions of higher education with health professions programs should seek opportunities to collaborate with neighboring school districts through public health initiatives that serve to mitigate vaccine mis- and disinformation and mistrust. Combating this public health concern is a shared responsibility.

6.6 Conclusions

The abundance of medical misinformation and disinformation on the internet, particularly through social media, is a public health concern. Vaccine hesitancy exemplifies how myths and misperceptions driven by mis- and disinformation affect patient care and population health. Conversations about vaccine hesitancy promulgated by mis/disinformation are challenging but integral to encouraging high vaccination rates, which is important for patient and population health. Educating health occupations students through an interprofessional, team approach that utilizes simulation-based learning, team-based learning, gamification, or other active learning pedagogy such as virtual or augmented reality can equip them with the knowledge and skills they need to successfully navigate this topic upon entry into practice.

References

1. Allen N, Harden J. Parental decision-making in uptake of the MMR vaccination: a systematic review of qualitative literature. J Public Health. 2015;37(4):678–87. https://doi.org/10.1093/pubmed/fdu075.
2. Barton SM, Calhoun AW, Bohnert CA, et al. Standardized vaccine-hesitant patients in the assessment of the effectiveness of vaccine communication training. J Pediatr. 2022;241:203–11. https://doi.org/10.1016/j.jpeds.2021.10.033.
3. Best S, Beech C, Robbé IJ, Williams S. Interprofessional teamwork: the role of professional identity and signature pedagogy – a mixed methods study. J Health Organ Manag. 2021; ahead-of-print: https://doi.org/10.1108/JHOM-06-2020-0242.
4. Blakeney EA, Owen JA, Ottis E, et al. Measuring the Impact of the National Train-the-Trainer Interprofessional Team Development Program (T3-ITDP) on the Implementation of Interprofessional Education and Interprofessional Collaborative Practice. J Interprof Educ Pract. 2021;24:100442. https://doi.org/10.1016/j.xjep.2021.100442.
5. Brashier NM, Pennycook G, Berinsky AJ, Rand DG. Timing matters when correcting fake news. Proc Natl Acad Sci. 2021;118(5):e2020043118. https://doi.org/10.1073/pnas.2020043118.
6. Buhse M, Della RC. Enhancing interprofessional education with team-BASED learning. Nurse Educ. 2017;42(5):240–4. https://doi.org/10.1097/NNE.0000000000000370.
7. Burgess A, Roberts C, van Diggele C, Mellis C. Peer teacher training (PTT) program for health professional students: interprofessional and flipped learning. BMC Med Educ. 2017a;17(1):239. https://doi.org/10.1186/s12909-017-1037-6.
8. Burgess A, Bleasel J, Haq I, et al. Team-based learning (TBL) in the medical curriculum: better than PBL? BMC Med Educ. 2017b;17(1):243. https://doi.org/10.1186/s12909-017-1068-z.
9. Burgess A, van Diggele C, Mellis C. Faculty development for junior health professionals. Clin Teach. 2019;16(3):189–96. https://doi.org/10.1111/tct.12795.
10. Burgess A, van Diggele C, Matar E. Interprofessional team-based learning: building social capital. J Med Educat Curri Develop. 2020;7:2382120520941820. https://doi.org/10.1177/2382120520941820.
11. Campisi CA, Li EH, Jiminez DE, Milanaik RL. Augmented reality in medical education and training: from physicians to patients. In: Geroimenko V, editor. Augmented reality in education. Switzerland: Springer; 2020. p. 111–38.

12. Canadian Interprofessional Health Collaborative. A National Interprofessional Competency Framework. https://phabc.org/wp-content/uploads/2015/07/CIHC-National-Interprofessional-Competency-Framework.pdf. Accessed 12 Oct 2023.
13. Cerf VG. Information and Misinformation on the Internet. Communication of the Association for Computing Machinery 2017. https://cacm.acm.org/magazines/2017/1/211112-information-and-misinformation-on-the-internet/fulltext/. Accessed 10 Oct 2023.
14. Chou WS, Oh A, Klein WMP. Addressing health-related misinformation on social media. JAMA J Am Med Assoc. 2018;320(23):2417–8. https://doi.org/10.1001/jama.2018.16865.
15. Damaševičius R, Maskeliūnas R, Blažauskas T. Serious games and gamification in healthcare: a meta-review. Information. 2023;14(2):105. https://doi.org/10.3390/info14020105.
16. Davitadze M, Ooi E, Ng CY, et al. SIMBA: using Kolb's learning theory in simulation-based learning to improve participants' confidence. BMC Med Educ. 2022;22(1):116. https://doi.org/10.1186/s12909-022-03176-2.
17. Dearnley C, Rhodes C, Roberts P, Williams P, Prenton S. Team based learning in nursing and midwifery higher education; a systematic review of the evidence for change. Nurse Educ Today. 2018;60:75–83. https://doi.org/10.1016/j.nedt.2017.09.012.
18. Demircioglu T, Karakus M, Ucar S. Developing students' critical thinking skills and argumentation abilities through augmented reality–based argumentation activities in science classes. Sci Educ. 2023;32(4):1165–95. https://doi.org/10.1007/s11191-022-00369-5.
19. El Mikati IK, Hoteit R, Harb T, et al. Defining misinformation and related terms in health-related literature: scoping review. J Med Internet Res. 2023;25:e45731. https://doi.org/10.2196/45731.
20. Ericsson KA. Deliberate practice and the acquisition and maintenance of expert performance: a general overview. Acad Emerg Med. 2008;15(11):988–94. https://doi.org/10.1111/j.1553-2712.2008.00227.x.
21. Fewster-Thuente L, Batteson TJ. Kolb's experiential learning theory as a theoretical underpinning for interprofessional education. J Allied Health. 2018;47(1):3–8.
22. Foltz-Ramos K, Fusco NM, Paige JB. Saving patient x: a quasi-experimental study of teamwork and performance in simulation following an interprofessional escape room. J Interprof Care. 2021:1–8. https://doi.org/10.1080/13561820.2021.1874316.
23. Fox L, Onders R, Hermansen-Kobulnicky CJ, et al. Teaching interprofessional teamwork skills to health professional students: a scoping review. J Interprof Care. 2018;32(2):127–35. https://doi.org/10.1080/13561820.2017.1399868.
24. Frederickson DD, Davis TC, Arnold CL, et al. Childhood immunization refusal: provider and parent perceptions. Fam Med. 2004;36(6):431–9.
25. Freed GL, Clark SJ, Butchart AT, et al. Parental vaccine safety concerns in 2009. Pediatrics. 2010;125(4):654–9. https://doi.org/10.1542/peds.2009-1962.
26. Freed GL, Clark SJ, Butchart AT, et al. Sources and perceived credibility of vaccine-safety information for parents. Pediatrics. 2011;127(Suppl 1):S107–12. https://doi.org/10.1542/peds.2010-1722P.
27. Friedrich C, Teaford H, Taubenheim A, Boland P, Sick B. Escaping the professional silo: an escape room implemented in an interprofessional education curriculum. J Interprof Care. 2019;33(5):573–5. https://doi.org/10.1080/13561820.2018.1538941.
28. Friedrich C, Teaford H, Taubenheim A, Sick B. Interprofessional health care escape room for advanced learners. J Nurs Educ. 2020;59(1):46–50. https://doi.org/10.3928/01484834-20191223-11.
29. Fusco NM, Foltz-Ramos K. Measuring changes in pharmacy and nursing students' perceptions following an interprofessional high-fidelity simulation experience. J Interprof Care. 2018;32(5):648–52. https://doi.org/10.1080/13561820.2018.1496073.
30. Fusco NM, Jacobsen LJ, Klem N, Krzyzanowicz R, Ohtake PJ. A serious game employed to introduce principles of interprofessional collaboration to students of multiple health professions. Simul Gaming. 2022a;53(3):253–64. https://doi.org/10.1177/10468781221093816.

31. Fusco NM, Foltz-Ramos K, Ohtake PJ. An interprofessional escape room experience to improve knowledge and collaboration among health professions students. Am J Pharm Educ. 2022b;86(9):8823. https://doi.org/10.5688/ajpe8823.
32. Fusco NM, Foltz-Ramos K, Kruger JS, Vargovich A, Prescott WA Jr. Interprofessional simulation to prepare students to address medical misinformation and vaccine hesitancy. J Interprof Educ Pract. 2023a;32:100644. https://doi.org/10.1016/j.xjep.2023.100644.
33. Fusco NM, Foltz-Ramos K, Zhao Y, Ohtake PJ. Virtual escape room paired with simulation improves health professions students' readiness to function in interprofessional teams. Curr Pharm Teach Learn. 2023b;15(3):311–8. https://doi.org/10.1016/j.cptl.2023.03.011.
34. Gallup®. Nurses Retain Top Ethics Rating in U.S., but Below 2020 High. https://news.gallup.com/poll/467804/nurses-retain-top-ethics-rating-below-2020-high.aspx. Accessed 20 Oct 2023.
35. Goldie J. The formation of professional identity in medical students: considerations for educators. Med Teach. 2012;34(9):e641–8. https://doi.org/10.3109/0142159X.2012.687476.
36. Health Professions Accreditors Collaborative (HPAC). IPE Guidance. https://healthprofessionsaccreditors.org/ipe-guidance/. Accessed 13 Oct 2023.
37. Hean S, Green C, Anderson E, et al. The contribution of theory to the design, delivery, and evaluation of interprofessional curricula: BEME Guide No. 49. Med Teach. 2018;40(6):542–58. https://doi.org/10.1080/0142159X.2018.1432851.
38. Helbing RR, Lapka S, Richdale K, Hatfield CL. In-person and online escape rooms for individual and team-based learning in health professions library instruction. J Med Libr Assoc. 2022;110(4):507–12. https://doi.org/10.5195/jmla.2022.1463.
39. History of Vaccines: History of Anti-Vaccination Movements. https://historyofvaccines.org/vaccines-101/misconceptions-about-vaccines/history-anti-vaccination-movements. Accessed 9/6/2024.
40. Hodges BD, Kuper A. Theory and practice in the design and conduct of graduate medical education. Acad Med. 2012;87(1):25–33. https://doi.org/10.1097/ACM.0b013e318238e069.
41. Homeyer S, Hoffmann W, Hingst P, Oppermann RF, Dreier-Wolfgramm A. Effects of interprofessional education for medical and nursing students: enablers, barriers and expectations for optimizing future interprofessional collaboration – a qualitative study. BMC Nurs. 2018;17:13. https://doi.org/10.1186/s12912-018-0279-x.
42. Hough-Telford C, Kimberlin DW, Aban I, et al. Vaccine delays, refusals, and patient dismissals: a survey of pediatricians. Pediatrics. 2016;138(3):e20162127. https://doi.org/10.1542/peds.2016-2127.
43. Hughes AM. Human factors in healthcare: theoretical underpinnings for simulation in interprofessional education. In: Levine A, DeMaria S, editors. Comprehensive healthcare simulation. Switzerland: Springer; 2020. p. 33–47.
44. Hursman A, Richter LM, Frenzel J, Viets Nice J, Monson E. An online escape room used to support the growth of teamwork in health professions students. J Interprof Educ Pract. 2022;29:100545. https://doi.org/10.1016/j.xjep.2022.100545.
45. INACSL Standards Committee. Healthcare Simulation Standards of Best Practice ™. Clin Simul Nurs. 2021;58:66. https://doi.org/10.1016/j.ecns.2021.08.018.
46. Institute of Medicine. Strengthening the Evidence Base. In: Briere R, editor. Measuring the impact of interprofessional education on collaborative practice and patient outcomes. 1st ed. Washington, DC: The National Academies Press; 2015. p. 39–49.
47. Interprofessional Education Collaborative (IPEC). IPEC Core Competencies Revision: Version 3. Washington, DC: Interprofessional Education Collaborative. https://www.ipecollaborative.org/2021-2023-core-competencies-revision. Accessed 6 Sept 2024.
48. Itin CM. Reasserting the philosophy of experiential education as a vehicle for change in the 21st century. J Exp Educ. 1999;22(2):91–8. https://doi.org/10.1177/105382599902200206.
49. James S, Cogan P, McCollum M. Team-based learning for immunology courses in allied health programs. Front Immunol. 2019;10:2477. https://doi.org/10.3389/fimmu.2019.02477.

50. Joseph S, Diack L. Playing interprofessional games: reflections on using the Interprofessional Education Game (iPEG). J Interprof Care. 2015;29(3):260–2. https://doi.org/10.3109/13561820.2014.942839.
51. Joshi T, Budhathoki P, Adhikari A, Poudel A, Raut S, Shrestha DB. Team-based learning among health care professionals: a systematic review. Cureus. 2022;14(1):e21252. https://doi.org/10.7759/cureus.21252.
52. Jung Y. Virtual reality simulation for disaster preparedness training in hospitals: integrated review. J Med Internet Res. 2022;24(1):e30600. https://doi.org/10.2196/30600.
53. Kennedy AM, Brown CJ, Gust DA. Vaccine beliefs of parents who oppose compulsory vaccination. Public Health Rep. 2005;120(3):252–8. https://doi.org/10.1177/003335490512000306.
54. Khullar D. Social media and medical misinformation: confronting new variants of an old problem. JAMA J Am Med Assoc. 2022;328(14):1393–4. https://doi.org/10.1001/jama.2022.17191.
55. Kolb D. Experiential learning: Experience as the source of learning and development. Engle Wood Cliffs and NJ: Prentice Hall; 1984.
56. Kugler AJ, Gogineni HP, Garavalia LS. Learning outcomes and student preferences with flipped vs lecture/case teaching model in a block curriculum. Am J Pharm Educ. 2019;83(8):7044. https://doi.org/10.5688/ajpe7044.
57. Kumar P, Paton C, Simpson HM, King CM, McGowan N. Is interprofessional co-debriefing necessary for effective interprofessional learning within simulation-based education? Int J Healthc Simul. 2021;1(1):49–55. https://doi.org/10.54531/INRX6536.
58. Lackie K, Hayward K, Ayn C, Stilwell P, Lane J, Andrews C, Dutton T, Ferkol D, Harris J, Houk S, Pendergast N. Creating psychological safety in interprofessional simulation for health professional learners: a scoping review of the barriers and enablers. J Interprof Care. 2023;37(2):187–202. https://doi.org/10.1080/13561820.2022.2052269.
59. Lapierre A, Lavoie P, Castonguay V, Lonergan AM, Arbour C. The influence of the simulation environment on teamwork and cognitive load in novice trauma professionals at the emergency department: Piloting a randomized controlled trial. Int Emerg Nurs. 2023;67:101261. https://doi.org/10.1016/j.ienj.2022.101261.
60. Larson HJ. The biggest pandemic risk? Viral misinformation. Nature. 2018;562(7726):309–10. https://doi.org/10.1038/d41586-018-07034-4.
61. Lein DH Jr, Lowman JD, Eidson CA, Yuen HK. Evaluation of team-based learning in a doctor of physical therapy curriculum in the United States. J Educ Eval Health Prof. 2017;14:3. https://doi.org/10.3352/jeehp.2017.14.3.
62. Luctkar-Flude M, Tyerman J, Tregunno D, et al. Designing a virtual simulation game as presimulation preparation for a respiratory distress simulation for senior nursing students: usability, feasibility, and perceived impact on learning. Clin Simul Nurs. 2021;52:35–42. https://doi.org/10.1016/j.ecns.2020.11.009.
63. MacDonald NE, the SAGE Working Group on Vaccine Hesitancy. Vaccine hesitancy: definition, scope and determinants. Vaccine. 2015;33(34):4161–4. https://doi.org/10.1016/j.vaccine.2015.04.036.
64. Maddock B, Dārziņš P, Kent F. Realist review of interprofessional education for health care students: What works for whom and why. J Interprof Care. 2023;37(2):173–86. https://doi.org/10.1080/13561820.2022.2039105.
65. Magill M, Hallgren KA. Mechanisms of behavior change in motivational interviewing: do we understand how MI works? Curr Opin Psychol. 2019;30:1–5. https://doi.org/10.1016/j.copsyc.2018.12.010.
66. Miller WR, Rollnick S. Motivational interviewing: Helping people change. 3rd ed. New York: Guilford press; 2012. p. 14–6.
67. National Center for Interprofessional Practice and Education. https://nexusipe.org/. Accessed 13 Oct 2023.

68. Nishigawa K, Omoto K, Hayama R, et al. Comparison between flipped classroom and team-based learning in fixed prosthodontic education. J Prosthodont Res. 2017;61(2):217–22. https://doi.org/10.1016/j.jpor.2016.04.003.
69. Office of the Surgeon G. Publications and Reports of the Surgeon General. Confronting Health Misinformation: The US Surgeon General's Advisory on Building a Healthy Information Environment 2021. https://www.hhs.gov/sites/default/files/surgeon-general-misinformation-advisory.pdf. Accessed 20 Oct 2023.
70. Ofstad W, Brunner LJ. Team-based learning in pharmacy education. Am J Pharm Educ. 2013;77(4):70. https://doi.org/10.5688/ajpe77470.
71. O'Neil-Pirozzi TM, Musler JL, Carney M, et al. Impact of early implementation of experiential education on the development of interprofessional education knowledge and skill competencies. J Allied Health. 2019;48(2):e53E–e9.
72. Paas FG, Van Merriënboer JJ, Adam JJ. Measurement of cognitive load in instructional research. Percept Mot Skills. 1994;79(1):419–30. https://doi.org/10.2466/pms.1994.79.1.419.
73. Paas F, Renkl A, Sweller J. Cognitive load theory and instructional design: recent developments. Educ Psychol. 2003;38(1):1–4. https://doi.org/10.1207/S15326985EP3801_1.
74. Paige JT, Garbee DD, Yu Q, et al. Brick in the wall? Linking quality of debriefing to participant learning in team training of interprofessional students. BMJ Simul Technol Enhanc Learn. 2021;7(5):360–5. https://doi.org/10.1136/bmjstel-2020-000685.
75. Poore JA, Cullen DL, Schaar GL. Simulation-based interprofessional education guided by Kolb's experiential learning theory. Clin Simul Nurs. 2014;10(5):e241–7. https://doi.org/10.1016/J.ECNS.2014.01.004.
76. Prescott WA Jr, Woodruff A, Prescott GM, et al. Introduction and assessment of a blended-learning model to teach patient assessment in a doctor of pharmacy program. Am J Pharm Educ. 2016;80(10):176. https://doi.org/10.5688/ajpe8010176.
77. Prescott WA Jr. Advanced pediatric therapeutics. In: Eiland LS, editor. Immunization controversies in children. 2nd ed. East Dundee: Pediatric Pharmacy Association; 2023. p. 374–82.
78. Prothero A. EducationWeek. Many Schools Don't Teach About the Science of Vaccines. Here's Why They Should. 2021. https://www.edweek.org/teaching-learning/many-schools-dont-teach-about-the-science-of-vaccines-heres-why-they-should/2021/07. Accessed 12 Oct 2023.
79. Puri N, Coomes EA, Haghbayan H, Gunaratne K. Social media and vaccine hesitancy: new updates for the era of COVID-19 and globalized infectious diseases. Hum Vaccin Immunother. 2020;16(11):2586–93. https://doi.org/10.1080/21645515.2020.1780846.
80. Real FJ, DeBlasio D, Beck AF, et al. A virtual reality curriculum for pediatric residents decreases rates of influenza vaccine refusal. Acad Pediatr. 2017;17(4):431–5. https://doi.org/10.1016/j.acap.2017.01.010.
81. Real FJ, Ollberding NJ, Meisman AR, et al. Impact of a virtual reality curriculum on human papillomavirus vaccination: a pilot trial. Am J Prev Med. 2022;63(5):865–73. https://doi.org/10.1016/j.amepre.2022.05.003.
82. Reeves S, Perrier L, Goldman J, Freeth D, Zwarenstein M. Interprofessional education: effects on professional practice and healthcare outcomes (update). Cochrane Database Syst Rev. 2013;2013(3):CD002213. https://doi.org/10.1002/14651858.CD002213.pub3.
83. Rogers BA, Franklin AE. Cognitive load experienced by nurses in simulation-based learning experiences: an integrative review. Nurse Educ Today. 2021;99:104815. https://doi.org/10.1016/j.nedt.2021.104815.
84. Rosen MA, DiazGranados D, Dietz AS, et al. Teamwork in healthcare: key discoveries enabling safer, high-quality care. Am Psychol. 2018;73(4):433–50. https://doi.org/10.1037/amp0000298.
85. Ruiz MG, Ezer H, Purden M. Exploring the nature of facilitating interprofessional learning: findings from an exploratory study. J Interprof Care. 2013;27(6):489–95. https://doi.org/10.3109/13561820.2013.811640.

86. Salmon DA, Moulton LH, Omer SB, et al. Factors associated with refusal of childhood vaccines among parents of school-aged children. Arch Pediatr Adolesc Med. 2005;159(5):470–6. https://doi.org/10.1001/archpedi.159.5.470.
87. Scales D, Gorman JM, DiCaprio P, et al. Community-oriented Motivational Interviewing (MI): A novel framework extending MI to address COVID-19 vaccine misinformation in online social media platforms. Comput Hum Behav. 2023;141:107609. https://doi.org/10.1016/j.chb.2022.107609.
88. Shrader S, Farland MZ, Danielson J, Sicat B, Umland EM. A systematic review of assessment tools measuring interprofessional education outcomes relevant to pharmacy education. Am J Pharm Educ. 2017;81(6):119. https://doi.org/10.5688/ajpe816119.
89. Sourg HAA, Satti S, Ahmed N, Ahmed ABM. Impact of flipped classroom model in increasing the achievement for medical students. BMC Med Educ. 2023;23(1):287. https://doi.org/10.1186/s12909-023-04276-3.
90. Suh I, McKinney T, Siu KC. Current perspective of metaverse application in medical education, research and patient care. Virtual Worlds. 2023;2(2):115–28. https://doi.org/10.3390/virtualworlds2020007.
91. Sweller J. Cognitive load theory, learning difficulty, and instructional design. Learn Instruct. 1994;4(4):295–312. https://doi.org/10.1016/0959-4752(94)90003-5.
92. The Vaccine Makers Project. https://vaccinemakers.org/. Accessed 12 Oct 2023.
93. Turkelson C, Yorke AM, Keiser M, Smith L, Gilbert GE. Promoting interprofessional communication with virtual simulation and deliberate practice. Clin Simul Nurs. 2020;46:30–9. https://doi.org/10.1016/j.ecns.2020.03.008.
94. Tyerman J, Luctkar-Flude M, Chumbley L, et al. Developing virtual simulation games for presimulation preparation: a user-friendly approach for nurse educators. J Nurs Educ Pract. 2021;11(7):10–8. https://doi.org/10.1016/j.ecns.2020.11.009.
95. United Nations Children's Fund (UNICEF). Interpersonal Communication for Immunization Training for Front Line Workers. https://www.unicef.org/eca/media/8576/file/interpersonal-communication-participant.pdf. Accessed 20 Oct 2023.
96. University of California San Francisco. Program for Interprofessional Practice and Education: Framework & Competencies. https://interprofessional.ucsf.edu/framework-competencies. Accessed 13 Oct 2023.
97. van Gaalen AEJ, Brouwer J, Schönrock-Adema J, et al. Gamification of health professions education: a systematic review. Adv Health Sci Educ Theory Pract. 2021;26(2):683–711. https://doi.org/10.1007/s10459-020-10000-3.
98. Wang JM, Zorek JA. Deliberate practice as a theoretical framework for interprofessional experiential education. Front Pharmacol. 2016;7:188. https://doi.org/10.3389/fphar.2016.00188.
99. Ward W, Zagoloff A, Rieck C, Robiner W. Interprofessional education: opportunities and challenges for psychology. J Clin Psychol Med Settings. 2018;25(3):250–66. https://doi.org/10.1007/s10880-017-9538-3.
100. Watt-Watson J, Hunter J, Pennefather P, et al. An integrated undergraduate pain curriculum, based on IASP curricula, for six health science faculties. Pain. 2004;110(1–2):140–8. https://doi.org/10.1016/j.pain.2004.03.019.
101. West C, Graham L, Palmer RT, et al. Implementation of interprofessional education (IPE) in 16 U.S. medical schools: Common practices, barriers and facilitators. J Interprof Educ Pract. 2016;4:41–9. https://doi.org/10.1016/j.xjep.2016.05.002.
102. Wong PS, Chen YS, Saw PS. Influencing factors and processes of interprofessional professional education (IPE) implementation. Med Teach. 2021;43(Suppl 1):S39–45. https://doi.org/10.1080/0142159X.2019.1672864.
103. Wong JY, Ko J, Nam S, et al. Virtual ER, a serious game for interprofessional education to enhance teamwork in medical and nursing undergraduates: development and evaluation study. JMIR Serious Games. 2022;10(3):e35269. https://doi.org/10.2196/35269.

104. World Health Organization. Ten Threats to global health in 2019. https://www.who.int/newsroom/spotlight/ten-threats-to-global-health-in-2019. Accessed 20 Oct 2023.
105. World Health Organization. Framework for action on interprofessional education & collaborative practice. https://www.who.int/publications/i/item/framework-for-action-on-interprofessional-education-collaborative-practice. Accessed 18 Oct 2023.
106. Yorke AM, Hoelscher DC, Stalburg CM, et al. Interprofessional education faculty development survey: perspectives on IPE and collaborative practice and COVID-19. J Interprof Educ Pract. 2022;29:100529. https://doi.org/10.1016/j.xjep.2022.100529.
107. Zorek JA, Ragucci K, Eickhoff J, et al. Development and validation of the IPEC Institutional Assessment Instrument. J Interprof Educ Pract. 2022;29:100553. https://doi.org/10.1016/j.xjep.2022.100553.

Chapter 7
Motivational Interviewing

Kayla Lauffer, Alec Harrington, Luke Twenhafel, Anicka Gajar, William Kang, Sharon Ke, Aleesa Rosas, Kyle Wansing, Gianna Tarka, and Benjamin Brooks

7.1 Introducing Motivational Interviewing and Vaccine Hesitancy

Motivational Interviewing (MI), a highly effective and patient-centered therapeutic technique, was developed initially by clinical psychologists William R. Miller and Stephen Rollnick in the 1980s [1]. Widely used in various fields including primary care professions, addiction treatment, and counseling, MI helps individuals explore and resolve ambivalence about behavioral change [2]. At its core, MI adopts a collaborative and empathetic approach, recognizing the importance of an individual's intrinsic motivation for change. MI has been found to be effective when individuals have the desire to change certain behaviors attributed to the quality of their lives, such as overcoming sexual addiction, engaging in smoking cessation, managing weight, adhering to medications, and addressing mental health concerns [3, 4]. While the outcomes may change, these individuals may still express competing desires and fears that create ambivalence resulting in an inability to make changes toward the desired behavior [5].

When the word "intervention" is mentioned, it often conjures images of individuals walking into an emotionally charged room with their loved ones seated in a circle. However, interventions take many forms, with MI being one of them [6]. MI allows for a gentle approach to addressing a person's behaviors due to its emphasis

K. Lauffer · A. Harrington · L. Twenhafel · A. Gajar · W. Kang · S. Ke · A. Rosas
K. Wansing · G. Tarka
College of Osteopathic Medicine, Rocky Vista University, Englewood, CO, USA

B. Brooks (✉)
College of Osteopathic Medicine, Rocky Vista University, Englewood, CO, USA

Department of Biomedical Sciences, Rocky Vista University, Ivins, UT, USA
e-mail: bbrooks@rvu.edu

A. J. Chase et al. (eds.), *Vaccine Hesitancy Curriculum*,
https://doi.org/10.1007/978-3-031-88668-3_7

on self-driven change. Notably, trained professionals are not exclusive users of this technique; it is accessible for anyone to use. This accessibility makes it an effective tool for interpersonal interventions. Couples, family members, friends, and even roommates can benefit from the ability to prompt change. MI proves to be a versatile tool in various interpersonal settings including vaccine promotion [7, 8].

Vaccine Hesitancy (VH) as a phenomenon is generally characterized as a behavior associated with the acceptance of some vaccines and the denial of others leading to the delay or acceptance of vaccines according to a recommended schedule [9]. The emergence of VH in the post-COVID pandemic era presents a complex challenge to global health. Amid the backdrop of rapidly developed vaccines, a portion of the population is reluctant to participate in vaccination programs, driven by concerns over efficacy and safety. This hesitancy has profound implications, potentially stalling the collective march toward herd immunity and re-establishing regular social and community activities amid evolving variants, considering the challenges of VH [10]. In confronting this issue, the medical community emphasizes the importance of transparent vaccine research and development process dissemination [6]. The focus is reinforcing public trust through evidence-based dialogue, addressing misinformation, and highlighting the rigorous scientific scrutiny underpinning vaccine approvals. Educational campaigns are tailored to resonate across diverse demographics, employing culturally competent messaging to reach and reassure skeptical groups [11]. These challenges provide an opportunity to use MI for VH [8].

In using MI for VH, practitioners observe a discernible shift in patients' readiness to consider vaccination, highlighting the technique's potency in transforming reluctance into acceptance [8]. Using MI in the VH realm has yielded promising results, substantiating the significance of use in public health endeavors, especially important with the current escalation of VH [12]. The MI process starts with active listening, which catalyzes a trusting relationship crucial for engaging patients in a dialogue about vaccination. The importance of MI transcends mere conversation, as it actively engages patients in a process that respects their autonomy and personal health philosophies, bridging the gap between hesitancy and trust. Studies show that when patients perceive the decision to vaccinate as emerging from their values and reasoning, facilitated by the MI process, their commitment to vaccination increases [12, 13]. In the planning phase of MI, the collaborative design of action plans further cements patients' resolve, indicating a direct correlation between MI engagement and improved vaccination rates. This discussion elaborates on the background, rationale, and elements for using MI as a tool, enabling healthcare professionals to navigate the nuanced landscape of patients with VH [12].

A key aspect of conducting MI is the environment in which it is performed. The interviewer must provide empathy, demonstrating reflective listening, genuineness, and warmth [14]. Under these conditions, the interviewer can have greater success using MI. This success is often reflected in the interviewee openly addressing their emotions and feelings toward the subject matter. For example, a patient seeing a practitioner with health concerns brought about by excessive alcohol consumption may not have entered the office ready to acknowledge a problem. However, with MI, the patient may feel safe enough to discuss that it has become a harmful habit and that this realization upsets them. In this example, MI enables patients to transition from denial to acknowledging their alcohol use disorder and their emotions toward that addiction. Furthermore, MI can be conducted to facilitate further progress as it allows the patient to recognize their feelings toward the subject and be open with themselves and the interviewer [15].

7.1.1 Cognitive Foundations in Motivational Interviewing: What Happens in Ambivalence?

MI is grounded in recognizing that patients often experience ambivalence, which is understood as conflicting feelings regarding a desired behavioral change. When one is at a crossroads for choices, decisions, or even emotions, ambivalence commonly follows [5]. Moving forward from ambivalence is critical, and many individuals can be stewards of promoting progression through the conflict of each side. Many people have unconsciously utilized this by considering the pros and cons, but the medical setting is beginning to implement its use. The goal is not to persuade a patient into one decision or another but to resolve ambivalence and move in the direction of change. Interviewers can utilize this tool to help their patients address topics they have been undecided on and then be able to provide treatment in harmony with the patient's values [5]. Take the earlier example of a patient with alcohol use disorder. This patient may have conflicting feelings about going sober. On the one hand, alcohol relaxes them and allows them a social outlet with friends; on the other, it negatively impacts their health and long-term relationships. They feel ambivalent about whether to continue drinking or to stop. MI allows the patient to analyze their values and decide what to do.

What follows the resolution of ambivalence? The patient has decided how they feel about a topic or what direction to take regarding it. So now what? Now, they must act. Aligning the behavior with the individual's values requires active effort. It is not easy to begin or maintain. As the founders of MI described, motivation to change comes from importance and confidence [5]. Resolving ambivalence has helped the person find what is important to them, but they must also be confident that they can successfully achieve change. Yet again, this is an opportunity for MI. Once confidence is built, assuming it is not already strong, the interviewer can begin helping the individual make behavioral changes that match their values. Returning to our patients with alcohol use disorder, assuming they chose to stop drinking, the interviewer can use MI to help the patient set reasonable goals for themself. Starting with small yet achievable goals like reducing the number of drinks per day by two can help build momentum for larger goals. This can empower the patient to continue making positive changes.

7.2 The Four Cardinal Principles of Conducting Motivational Interviewing

Before learning and practicing MI, one should understand the principles and overall spirit of the technique. MI supports patient autonomy using a collaborative approach to invoke the desire for change. Here, we will discuss the four principles of MI: express empathy, develop discrepancy, roll with resistance, and support self-efficacy [16, 17].

The first principle of MI is expressing empathy. The professional conversation between interviewer and patient is empathetic and patient-centered [16, 17]. Achieved through an accepting attitude and reflective listening, the interviewer aims to comprehend the patient's feelings and perspectives without judgment or blame. Such acceptance fosters ambivalence, thereby facilitating an opportunity for change. In contrast, judgmental and nonaccepting interactions can deter the patient and impede the change process. Key to expressing empathy in MI is understanding that acceptance promotes change, employing skillful reflective listening is crucial, and recognizing that ambivalence is a normal part of the process [16, 17].

Following the principle of expressing empathy is the development of discrepancy [16, 17]. The principle emerges naturally from empathetic conversations, wherein a discrepancy between the patient's current actions and their beliefs and values is highlighted, as seen from the patient's perspective. When a conflict arises between an individual's behavior and their goals, catalyzing change is possible. The conversational approach should enable patients to discover their reasons for change rather than being directed by the interviewer. Patients are typically more motivated to change when they articulate these reasons themselves rather than hearing them from someone else [5, 18]. The interviewer can then reinforce the patient's realization by verbally reflecting on the conclusions made. The cornerstone of developing discrepancy is understanding that the perceived gap between current behavior and significant personal goals or values drives change. The patient, not the interviewer, should articulate the arguments for change [18].

The following principle in MI is rolling with resistance. It is crucial to avoid advocating or pushing for change when a patient opposes it. Doing so might lead the patient further away from the desired change [16–18]. Instead, the interviewer should "roll with it" or adapt when faced with resistance. Altering the conversational approach in response to the patient's reluctance or resistance is involved. Presenting new information and perspectives can be beneficial in such scenarios. When rolling with resistance, clinical educators have a role in guiding the patient interaction using key strategies such as avoiding arguments for change, not directly confronting resistance, and welcoming new perspectives [19]. The patient is seen as a primary source for finding answers or solutions, and their resistance is viewed as a cue for the interviewer to adapt their response [16, 17].

The final principle of MI is supporting self-efficacy, which is crucial for change. Self-efficacy, a person's belief in their ability to succeed in tasks, can predict the outcome of change [16, 17]. This is encouraged by celebrating small victories

Table 7.1 Example phrases for each MI principle reflected in the literature of MI produced by Treasure 2004 [16]

MI principle	Example phrases for VH
Express empathy	"It is completely understandable to have concerns about new vaccines."
	"Many people feel uneasy about medical decisions; it is normal to have questions."
Develop discrepancy	"How do your concerns about vaccine safety align with your wish to stay healthy and protect your family?"
	"What are your thoughts on balancing the risks of the disease versus the risks of the vaccine?"
	"You mentioned you want to avoid getting sick; how does avoiding the vaccine fit that goal?"
Roll with resistance	"It seems like you have some strong reasons for being hesitant. Let's explore those a bit more."
	"I hear your concerns, and they're valid. What would make you feel more comfortable?"
	"Let's take a step back and consider the different perspectives on this issue."
Support self-efficacy	"I believe you can make the best decision for your health. What information do you feel you need to do that?"
	"You've made informed health decisions in the past; how might you apply that experience here?"
	"What steps would you feel comfortable taking to learn more about the vaccine?"

[16, 17]. This can be achieved with bi-weekly check-ins of a measurable outcome or utilizing parallel methods based on past success with behavior changes [16, 17]. Setting milestones can support self-efficacy and increase the chance of success with MI, with a counselor providing support along the way [16, 17]. If the client lacks hope or confidence in the possibility of change, motivation for change will be absent, and change will not occur. The client must believe in their capacity to implement change. By allowing the patient to take charge of conversations about change, the interviewer demonstrates faith in their abilities, which can become a self-fulfilling prophecy [16, 17] (Table 7.1).

7.3 Collaboration in Motivational Interviewing: Describing the Phases and Processes

In MI, the interviewer aims to create a nonjudgmental and supportive atmosphere where patients feel safe expressing their thoughts, concerns, and goals with success as demonstrated in challenges regarding medication adherence [20]. MI motivates people to make positive changes by exploring their reasons for change and perceived barriers to resolving ambivalence [16, 17]. MI involves active listening, reflective questioning, and guiding patients toward a deeper understanding of their values and aspirations. One of the central principles of MI is the belief that individuals are more likely to commit to change when they perceive it as their own choice rather than being pressured or coerced into making the lifestyle change [5].

The collaborative interaction seen in MI has been described in two phases: "Building Motivation for Change" and "Strengthening Commitment to Change" [5]. On reviewing these two phases, more recently, William Miller in 2023 stratifies these phases into four processes [18]. These processes are summarized as "Engaging, Focusing, Evoking, and Planning" [5, 18, 21, 22]. The first process of MI begins with "engaging" or building rapport with the interviewee [5, 14]. This first process establishes the collaborative relationship between the interviewer and the interviewee. By creating a supportive environment, the interviewer encourages interviewees to openly discuss their concerns and motivations for a potential change [7].

The second process of MI is "Focusing," which involves targeting specific behaviors that the patient wants to address [7, 14, 23]. This theme seeks to clarify the patient's goals and priorities in both the patient's and practitioner's eyes [14]. This theme requires the use of core interaction techniques found in MI known as "OARS": Open-ended questions, Affirmations, Reflective listening, and Summarizing [5].

The third process of MI is "Evoking," a process that explores the patient's motivations for change [14]. This process helps the patient better understand their motivations and ambivalence toward change. During the process of Evoking, open-ended questions and reflective listening as found in the OARS interaction techniques are vital as they elicit an individual's reasons for wanting to change [5, 14]. This process and the use of these tools are meant to emphasize the patient's autonomy and self-efficacy creating an invitation for them to consider their situation and find personal solutions to the identified problems [24].

The final process of MI is "Planning," which focuses on developing a personal commitment to change [14]. During "Planning," the interviewer collaborates with the patient to create a plan tailored to the patient's goals and preferences toward addressing a certain issue with efficiency, as reflected in the management of diabetes and obesity [14, 24]. As in the previous processes, the tools associated with OARS should be utilized throughout this process [14, 25].

7.4 The Importance of the Transtheoretical Model in Motivational Interviewing

MI was developed with evidence-based research to guide its format and processes. To achieve outcomes, individuals progress through the stages of change, these being pre-contemplation (not yet considering change), contemplation (considering change), preparation (getting ready to make change), taking action, and finally, maintenance (continuing the change long-term) [5]. This process of change is referred to as the Transtheoretical Model (TTM), which illustrates the various stages you may find someone in regarding lifestyle modifications and generally progressing through the stages sequentially [5]. The idea is to target intervention strategies based on the stage that someone is in to be most effective [26]. It is important to note that a person may begin this process at any stage and may regress. When someone is in the pre-contemplation stage, they have no perceived need or intention to change any future behavior. The switch to the contemplation stage occurs when people become aware of a potentially negative emotion such as regret resulting from a negative consequence that has occurred due to a committed action leading to a change in cognition toward making changes to maladaptive behaviors [27]. At this point, there is a lack of commitment to taking the steps necessary to accomplish the change. This transition is building readiness. Preparation is characterized by creating small behavioral and cognitive shifts required to put the desire for change into action [28]. Action is when a behavior change has been accomplished for a small amount of time [26, 28]. Maintenance occurs when the behavioral change persists in the long term [26, 28]. The maintenance phase also includes factors that prevent relapse and is where gains from the change are finally seen [27, 28].

Part of the interviewer's role in relation to the TTM is to determine which stage of change the person is in and act as a guide to move to the next step based on this model. However, it is essential to realize that this model is not all-inclusive, and everyone's cognition regarding motivations for behavior change is unique and may lead to the inability to follow the stages of the TTM sequentially [29]. Regardless, people do not like being told what to do, and MI, when done correctly based on the TTM, recognizes this. By establishing an environment with empathy, reflective listening, and genuineness from the interviewer, the individual is shown to respond far better [7, 30]. With MI being such a broad tool, it should be no surprise that many emerging models of its use exist and are continuing to be analyzed. However, despite the model used, it is imperative to recognize that motivations are unique to each person, and thus, growth and change must be chosen by that person. The individual conducting the interview guides the interviewee to introspect on their values and act accordingly. Because MI relies heavily on promoting autonomy, even within the framework of TTM, an interviewer can fail to utilize MI upon exerting an argument that is the opposite of the interviewee's opinion of what their emotions or progress is in changing behaviors [5, 26, 28].

7.5 OARS Interaction Techniques in the Setting of Motivational Interviewing

OARS (Open-ended questions, Affirmations, Reflective listening, and Summarizing) is a skills-based communication model that practitioners utilize heavily to effectively participate in MI [5, 8]. As suggested in the previous sections, practitioners aim to understand the patient's frame of reference, amplify statements encouraging change while dampening status quo statements, and elicit expressions demonstrating the patient's readiness to change. Matching processes used in MI theory to the patient's stage of change, the therapist expresses acceptance and affirmation of the patient's freedom of choice and self-direction regarding the change. Being flexible, practitioners balance acceptance and drive for change, suppressing any instincts to solve problems prematurely or directly set things right. MI's twofold goal is to increase the importance of change for the patient while bolstering their confidence that change can happen [16].

When participating in MI regardless of the process or model used to identify the patient's cognition toward a behavior, open-ended questions allow the patient to be involved in the conversation to facilitate a collaborative and empathetic therapeutic relationship [31]. Furthermore, open-ended questioning leads to greater information gathering as closed-questioning generally limits the conversation [32]. When open questions are asked, the recipient guides the conversation. This allows the time spent talking to be more equal between the two parties, ideally with the interviewer talking less than the patient [8].

Affirming entails encouraging strengths, thoughts, and actions that allow the patient to take steps toward healthy change [8]. People are more willing to self-reflect and change in a positive environment where they do not feel the need to defend themselves. Focusing on the helpful attributes of someone rather than their shortcomings can empower individuals, allowing for a shift in cognition that is more open and confident in their ability to be successful in change [8].

Reflection ensures that the patient feels heard and understood. The interviewer repeats and slightly rewords what has been said so that it becomes known that the information is not falling on deaf ears. Skillful reflection finds the balance between simply repeating what is being said and the other extreme of making exaggerated guesses and interpretations [8]. Instead, these skills can be considered reading between the lines and making connections that were not explicitly stated. These reflections should be expressed as statements.

Finally, summarizing creates a complete conversational picture. This allows the recipient's thoughts and motivations to be integrated cohesively, enabling the interviewer and the recipient to be on the same page. By implementing the acronym OARS, transparent and open communication can occur that welcomes the recipients' thoughts and facilitates their motivations to change to dominate the continuation of the conversation.

Using the OARS model provides a guideline to allow the practitioner and individual to identify and explore what motivations exist regarding behaviors and how they change to become the centerpiece and guiding notion of the conversation.

7.6 Motivational Interviewing Uses and Efficacy

While MI has been around for years, its uses continue to be investigated in situations spanning across different disciplines. MI is extensively applied and researched in various fields, including substance abuse, dental practice, primary care health professions, and mental health professions [15]. Initially envisioned and developed to address addiction, MI evolved from recognizing that direct persuasion is often ineffective in changing behavior, primarily due to the inability to resolve internal ambivalence [33]. In the mental health professions, MI continues to be used in managing conditions of addiction, substance abuse, and mental health disorders such as depression and anxiety by empowering patients to take active roles in their treatment [33, 34]. Furthermore, MI has extended to complement the treatment of conditions including eating disorders, post-traumatic stress disorder, obsessive-compulsive traits, and the initial refusal of psychiatric treatment with effectiveness [35].

Over time, the use of MI has expanded beyond the mental health professions to include fields such as primary care health professions and dental professions, where MI is used to encourage lifestyle changes such as smoking cessation, diet modification, and oral health behaviors with respect to both fields [15, 36]. Further effectiveness of MI based on a systematic review and meta-analysis on using MI with primary care populations demonstrates MI's ability in promoting behavioral change and improving health outcomes in blood pressure management, weight reduction, physical activity, and adherence when assessed together [37]. Furthermore, multiple studies demonstrate that MI helps patients address alcoholism, drug addiction, gambling, and even sex addiction by engaging patients to progress through stages of change and reduce self-destructive habits [1, 3, 38]. By understanding motivations and affirming self-efficacy, MI builds readiness and willingness to pursue recovery goals in modest steps or complete abstinence [1].

Within medical contexts, MI improves adherence to vital treatment protocols around medications, diet, exercise, and lifestyle changes. Beyond addiction populations, which are apparent groups for utilizing MI, there are less obvious groups benefiting from its implementation. Patients with chronic illness often struggle to maintain components of care essential to stability or prevention of decline [5]. This can be dangerous for patients who need to follow their treatment protocol to prevent adverse health events [5]. Aversion to adhering to prescribed treatment regimens can also worsen disease states beyond recovery. Because of this, MI is a tool that practitioners are being trained to use to help their patients choose to follow their treatments and improve health outcomes. By eliciting patient values and perspectives, MI gives practitioners tools to encourage commitment to treatment goals in patients managing health goals for things such as asthma, hypertension, or prenatal care [1, 3, 38]. Emphasizing patient autonomy and collaborative decision-making through MI strengthens the self-motivation and confidence needed to persist with complex treatment plans.

MI's effectiveness is demonstrated in various clinical trials and meta-analyses. Several controlled clinical trial meta-analyses found that MI effectively promoted behavior change [39–44]. A meta-analysis conducted by Burke et al. demonstrated MI for alcoholism to be more effective than placebo, leading to a 56% reduction in patient alcohol consumption [39]. Another meta-analysis conducted by Rubak et al. used clinical markers to empirically show the effectiveness of MI. Across multiple studies, MI led to a clinically significant decrease in associated markers such as body mass index, total blood cholesterol, systolic blood pressure, and blood alcohol concentration [39]. This meta-analysis also showed MI to be effective in studies on psychological (75% of studies) and physiological disease (72% of studies) [39]. In this study, MI was found to be effective in brief encounters. Also, 64% of studies found an effect after only 15 minutes of MI [39].

One of this tool's most recent and pertinent applications is to combat VH. As previously introduced, MI with VH has become the focus of emerging studies. Due in part to the attention given to VH in the context of parents and childhood vaccines, the studies that have emerged so far have been promising. These studies aimed to use MI to increase vaccine uptake and decrease VH in child patients. To benefit pediatric patients, physicians used MI techniques with parents to shift VH to acceptance with success [7, 45]. Another study investigated vaccination and MI efficacy with only one brief session. It followed infants for 3-, 5-, and 7-month-old vaccine reports. It found a significant increase in vaccination among the experimental group whose parents had received an individual MI session during their postpartum stay in the maternity ward [7].

7.7 Understanding Vaccine Hesitancy as a Spectrum

VH exists as a spectrum. This spectrum, illustrated in Fig. 7.1, extends from outright denial at one extreme to complete acceptance of all vaccines at the other [46]. The spectrum reflects individuals' diverse attitudes and beliefs, but a sociological component is often integrally woven into an individual's VH [46]. In this section, the VH spectrum sheds light on how MI techniques can be applied to different groups across the VH spectrum.

At one end of this spectrum, the vaccine deniers steadfastly and aggressively reject all vaccines, deny the scientific evidence supporting vaccines, and spread misinformation about vaccines. Moreover, they are unyielding in their opposition, and the denier label is often integrated into their worldview and that of their community. Vaccine denial is frequently based on deep-seated, ideologically driven

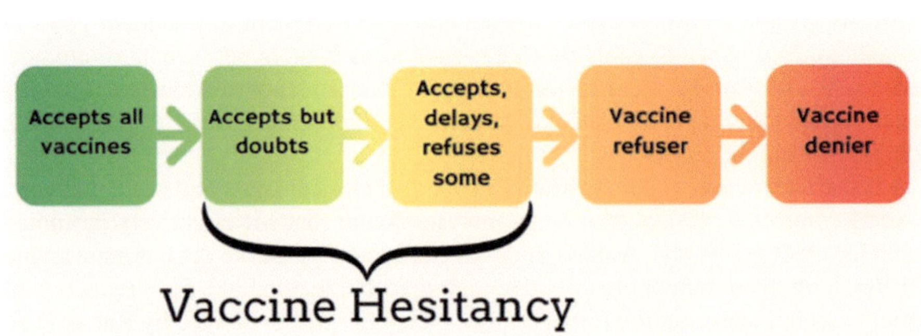

Fig. 7.1 Spectrum of VH, ranging from accepting all vaccines on the far left to denying all vaccines on the right. (The figure is adapted from Gill et al. (2022) and is inspired by the original spectrum of VH presented by Macdonald (2015) [46, 47])

misinformation or mistrust in scientific evidence and public health institutions. This group is often vocally strong and attempts to recruit others against vaccines. This group may be influenced by factors such as the experiences and opinions of trusted members of their community or a profound skepticism toward medical authority, leading to a categorical refusal of the safety and efficacy of all vaccines [46].

Progressing along the VH spectrum, vaccine refusers decline to receive most vaccines. Like deniers, this stance typically stems from deeply held beliefs or significant mistrust in the efficacy and safety of vaccines, often reinforced by misinformation or ideological biases. Various factors can influence their refusal, including personal or family health experiences, religious beliefs, or skepticism toward pharmaceutical companies and governmental health agencies. Vaccine refusers, while skeptical, generally base their reluctance on specific personal or spiritual beliefs. The primary difference between deniers and refusers is that the deniers reject the scientific consensus, whereas refusers are skeptical, and as such, deniers commonly spread misinformation aggressively [48].

The next group on the VH spectrum are those who are truly hesitant. This group is a nuanced and complex phenomenon often influenced by many personal, cultural, and psychological factors, leading to vaccine indecision [46]. This hesitancy can stem from concerns about potential side effects, doubts about the efficacy of vaccines, or mistrust in the healthcare system and pharmaceutical companies. The vaccine-hesitant individuals are also influenced by personal experiences, anecdotal accounts from others, and the broader social and media narratives surrounding vaccination. The dynamic nature of VH means that it can vary across time, place, and vaccines [46]. This group is somewhat open to vaccines but is reluctant. This group includes cautious acceptors who generally accept most vaccines but might have concerns ranging from ingredients, side effects, or the number of vaccines given at once [46].

At the other end of the spectrum are individuals that fully accept vaccines. This group trusts the scientific process behind their development and recognizes their crucial role in public health and disease prevention. This acceptance is usually grounded in comprehending vaccine safety profile efficacy data and appreciating the collective benefits of herd immunity or trust in medical authority [46, 49].

While this spectrum can be broadly applied to VH, it can also be used or modified for specific vaccines or scenarios as they arise. Plitch-Loeb et al. studied this spectrum regarding the COVID-19 vaccine as the vaccine became available in April 2022 [50]. Here, they used a very similar spectrum ranging from eagerness to take the vaccine/already vaccinated to outright refusal to examine the demographics of each group. In this study, the most relevant factors for those refusing or undecided on the vaccine were political affiliation and financial hardship experienced during the pandemic [50].

Regardless of where people may fall on the VH spectrum, it is important to realize that the behaviors individuals commit are not necessarily out of malice or disregard for themselves or others. Rather, the ability to rationalize these behaviors into beliefs or engage in social learning, while affected by adaptive processes such as cultural norms, societal pressures, and habits, is arguably meant to self-preserve the individual by avoiding stress secondary to cognitive strain and promote social fitness [51]. To explain briefly in detail using Fig. 7.2, the ability to rationalize behaviors and engage in social learning occurs in parallel when watching others engage in the behavior of interest and adapting said behavior followed by the learner making inferences about why they and their peers are engaging in said behavior [51].

VH, including the extremes of outright deniers, refusers, and those who accept all vaccines, can be intricately understood through the "5 Cs VH model": Confidence, Complacency, Convenience, Calculation, and Collective Responsibility (Fig. 7.3) [46, 49, 52]. Confidence refers to the trust in the vaccine's safety and efficacy and the system that creates and delivers the vaccines. Complacency happens when a belief develops that vaccination is unnecessary, usually when the perceived risks of vaccine-preventable diseases are low. Complacency can be due to the success of vaccines in controlling certain diseases, making them seem less of a threat. Constraints heavily influence VH, including access, affordability, and availability of vaccines. Calculation, defined as an individual weighing the perceived risks and benefits of vaccines, often is influenced by an overload of information and misinformation. Lastly, collective responsibility is an understanding of the role of vaccination in the broader public health context, where personal decisions impact community health [49].

For medical professionals, understanding and recognizing this spectrum and the associated 5Cs allows them to tailor a discussion based on the patient's VH level. This understanding also enables the practitioner to select the best communication strategies to address specific concerns and promote informed, health-positive decisions regarding vaccination.

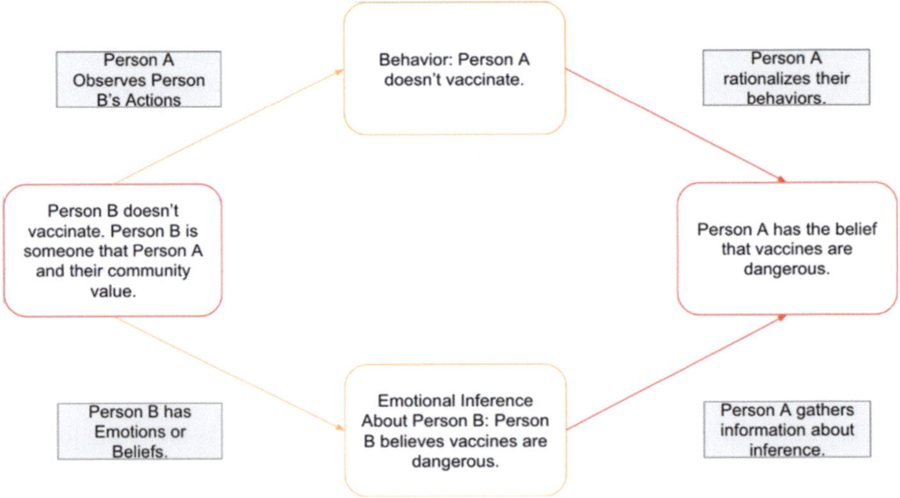

Fig. 7.2 Parallel pathways of social learning, as adapted from Cushman (2020), applied to developing VH behaviors [51]

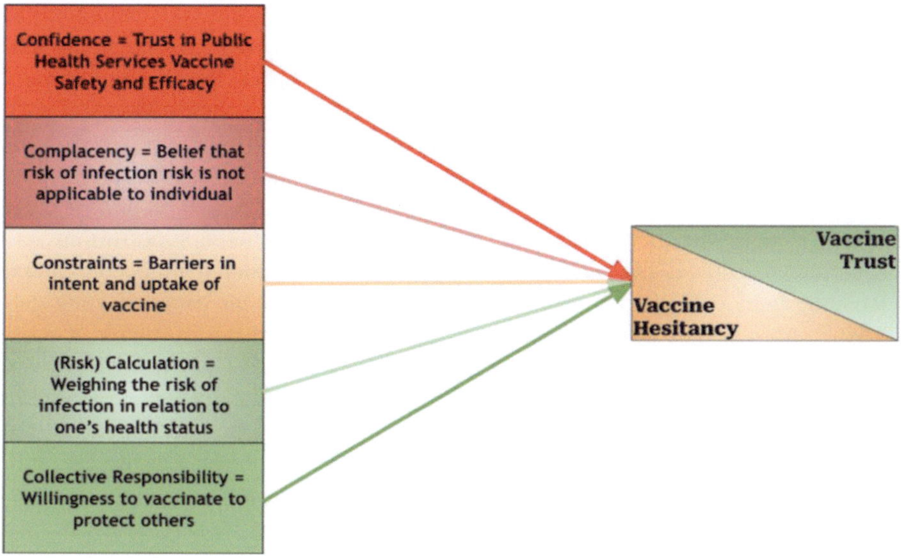

Fig. 7.3 The 5Cs VH Model adapted from Rancher et al. (2023) referencing the works of Betsch et al. (2018) [49]

7.7.1 The Vaccines Associated with Hesitancy

Some degree of VH exists for nearly every vaccine, but four common ones include COVID-19, HPV, MMR, and influenza [23, 53–55]. As mentioned previously, VH is a spectrum of behaviors that people engage in that can further influence their own beliefs or are adapted from other social and cultural pressures [51]. Some of these adaptive variables leading to hesitating about these vaccines have been previously given. However, regarding the four vaccines reported above, reported themes of knowledge of adverse effects, anecdotes from friends and family, lack of knowledge about vaccines, and personal superstitions may adapt to VH rationale [56].

Since the onset of the COVID-19 pandemic, there has been an increase in VH, and the public has become more interested in discussing their side effects. For example, the Vaccine Adverse Event Reporting System (VAERS) became a frequently used database in discussing vaccine safety, with the COVID-19 vaccine being frequently mentioned [57]. Various side effects have been reported, ranging from headache to death [57]. Since these entries are not extensively reviewed or audited, entries can be added by any public member without medical verification of direct causation. Therefore, if someone enters a severe adverse event, without verification, then the vaccine could appear to be dangerous to receive [57, 58]. Regardless of whoever is putting in data into VAERS, it cannot be denied that refusal of the COVID-19 vaccination is increasing as the rate of influenza vaccination also continues to decline [56, 59]. According to CDC data, the number of people saying they will "definitely or probably not get a vaccine" increased between the 2023–2024 season and the 2024–2025 season [59]. Furthermore, with measles beginning to increase in prevalence again in 2019, there has been a growing focus on parents who choose not to vaccinate their children [23, 56, 59, 60]. This presents an increasingly urgent need to find new ways to shift these parents' views of vaccination and push childhood vaccination rates toward herd immunity levels.

As previously discussed, VH is a social phenomenon that is multifaceted leading to possible root causes as to why someone engages in VH. In relation to how these factors relate to the mentioned vaccines above, look to shared superstitions and constructed narratives as a significant cause of VH. Specifically, it has been reported that some individuals perceive that the influenza vaccine is the cause for their getting influenza, despite the vaccine containing a killed virus that is incapable of causing active influenza infection [54]. Another belief is that if an HPV vaccine is given to a teenager, this teen is more likely to become sexually active despite research to the contrary [61]. The controversy around the MMR vaccine and autism started many decades ago; however, this concern has persisted into this decade [56, 60]. There have been many personal superstitions surrounding the COVID-19 vaccine, one being concern that people who are pro-vaccine are being hired by pharmaceutical companies to help sell their products [62].

Professionals in these fields may come across VH not only regarding newly developed vaccines but also in vaccines that have been used for years in vaccine schedules, leading to potential increases in morbidity and mortality. To further this point, it has been found that there has been a decreasing trend in adolescents within the United States acquiring the HPV vaccine, with the proportion of vaccinated children being well below the national goal of 80% vaccination along with VH of HPV predicted to be as high as 64% within the United States between 2019 and 2022 [63].

With the risk of infectious diseases, it is essential to acknowledge that individuals without contraindications for a preventable disease should, at the very least, receive appropriate information about the risks and complications associated with the decision to vaccinate. The risk of recurrence of these diseases may be minimal at this point. Still, the cost of treatment and mortality for some of these diseases cannot be disregarded, with management costs for vaccine-preventable diseases costing up to $27 billion annually [64]. However, these conversations are often difficult to have as professionals and patients can succumb to many challenges that appear in VH, such as communication within the appropriate patient context [65].

7.8 Applications of Motivational Interviewing in Vaccine Hesitancy

The fields most likely to see VH individuals will often be primary care-related, participating in ambulatory medicine. However, it cannot be denied that medical professionals may also come across VH in the hospital setting, as a study from Hofstetter et al. suggests that caregivers of hospitalized pediatric patients also present with VH and potential refusal of annual vaccines [66].

MI aims to enhance patients' motivation to modify their behavior based on their own reasoning, as well as support their decision-making process [67]. Central steps in MI are establishing relationship rapport, discussing specific behavior changes, and prioritizing the patient's genuine concerns [67]. In regard to vaccinations, MI's objective is to meet the patient on common ground, respect their beliefs, and cultivate a robust partnership, enabling empathetic and respectful discussions [67]. Various MI strategies are being explored and implemented to combat the rising problem of VH. The PromoVac Strategy, adopted in Quebec's maternity wards, exemplifies this [68]. A provincial randomized controlled trial reported a 40% decrease in VH scores using this strategy [69]. Dempsey et al. conducted a cluster randomized control trial in Denver, Colorado, testing a 5-component healthcare professional communication intervention based on the MI approach to increase HPV vaccinations. The intervention group had an 11.3% increase in initiating the vaccine compared to the 1.8% in the control group [70].

The foundation of any productive patient–practitioner relationship is trust, compassion, and acceptance [67]. Encounters with VH patients can backfire when patients are provided with only the facts and, even worse, with a subsequent condescending tone [67]. The first and most crucial step in MI with patients with VH is to take the time to foster a trusting partnership with patients. This step is essential in encouraging patients to share their experiences and concerns. This relationship can be built by emphasizing respect for the patient's autonomy and practicing with the patient's best interest in mind. Compassion includes actively listening to patients, meeting them at their level of knowledge, and involving them in health decisions. Acceptance entails maintaining a positive, empathetic attitude and creating a safe environment for patients to express their fears and queries. This approach can be effectively integrated into routine office visits like yearly physicals, well-child checks, and sick visits without focusing directly on the issue of VH.

During a session, the practitioner should foster engagement in patients with VH through the MI processes briefly discussed in a previous section: Engaging, Focusing, Evoking, and Planning [5, 14, 21, 22]. Engage the patient by showing empathy and genuine interest in their perspective on vaccines. Begin by setting an agenda focused on VH and inquire about the patient's understanding of vaccination and concerns. Focus the discussion solely on vaccinations, evaluating the patient's current knowledge and misconceptions. Evoke an open discussion by sharing resources and experiences and exploring the patient's reservations about vaccines. Plan for the future by discussing potential diseases preventable by vaccines, their symptoms, and prognoses so the patient can consider preventive actions. Lastly, keep VH an open topic for further discussion in subsequent visits. Table 7.2 provides examples of questions that can be asked in each of the phases of MI.

Table 7.2 Sample questions for each of the processes of MI adapted from Miller (2023) [14]

Phase	Sample questions
Engaging	
Set an agenda	How would you like to spend our time together today? What is your top priority right now?
Focusing	
Negotiation of focus	I hear you are concerned about your child's health. What are your thoughts about vaccines? At this 11-year-old well-child check, we administer HPV vaccines. Would you be open to receiving the shot today?
Scaling importance, confidence, and readiness	I would like to understand your thoughts and concerns on this topic. Would you be willing to learn more about this vaccine?
Evoking	
Importance of change	Here is my experience with vaccines and the diseases they protect against. Would you be willing to receive some of the vaccines protecting against the more concerning diseases? Would you be willing to work with me on an agreeable vaccine schedule?
Explore strengths	Was there a challenge you felt similar to hesitancy? What gave you the courage to overcome that challenge? What resources did you choose (family, friends, websites, books, social media)?
Planning	
Looking forward	What precautions have you taken to protect yourself or your child from potential diseases? Would you be open to continuing the discussion about this topic in future visits? How can we protect you from these potential diseases?

7.8.1 *The Challenges of Motivational Interviewing in Vaccine Hesitancy*

Despite the efficacy and uses of MI in VH and other situations, it is important to acknowledge that challenges such as spectrum identification, time, bias, and practitioner experience can have an impact on the use of MI in VH. The initial step of "spectrum identification" involves accurately identifying where the patient lies on the VH spectrum by inquiring about vaccines and gauging the response based on prior knowledge. Identifying where a patient is on the VH spectrum will significantly influence the practitioner's strategy in using MI. As discussed earlier, the VH continuum ranges from complete acceptance to outright refusal, with varying levels of hesitancy in between. Identifying the precise location of the patient within the VH continuum is critical because it shapes the practitioner's approach, tailoring interventions to match the patient's readiness to consider vaccination. For patients identified as refusers or deniers, setting expectations for immediate progress toward acceptance can be unrealistic and may lead to frustration on both sides [67]. This is mainly because, for people identified as vaccine refusers or deniers, their stance against vaccination is not merely an opinion but is often deeply entrenched in their identity. Such beliefs are core to who they are, making any challenge to these beliefs may feel like a personal attack [71]. Across time, change in perspective may occur;

however, progress may be slow or nonexistent, and the provider must be prepared for this scenario.

Furthermore, current and future practitioners must understand that the MI approach often requires multiple visits and should not be rushed in a single session. Meeting the patient where they are is crucial, prioritizing their health and wellness, regardless of their beliefs [5]. Developing trust may be the only prudent course. Fundamental to MI is establishing rapport and fostering a relationship that cannot be rushed, allowing patients to consider change, and respecting their autonomy and pace throughout the process. MI acknowledges the complexities of behavior change, advocating for a patient-centered strategy that values gradual progress over multiple sessions versus immediate results [5].

Additionally, a critical step for healthcare practitioners to tackle VH involves acknowledging and setting aside their biases. This process requires a conscious effort to identify and manage any personal prejudices or preconceived notions they may hold toward individuals with VH. By doing so, practitioners foster a nonjudgmental and supportive environment, which is paramount for effective patient engagement. Recognizing one's biases enhances the therapeutic relationship and ensures that medical care and advice are rooted in empathy and understanding rather than judgment. This commitment to impartiality helps build trust with the patient, a crucial element in guiding them toward making informed health decisions. Ultimately, approaching each patient's concerns with an open mind is essential for successfully navigating the complexities of VH [5].

Lastly, MI is heavily reliant on the practitioner's experience, emphasizing the need for a personal approach with every patient [72]. MI training should emphasize the importance of experiential learning and the expectation that progress will be achieved through a series of advances and setbacks. Consequently, the emphasis on allowing time for the practitioner's skill in MI to develop is beneficial and necessary for the implementation of MI to be truly impactful in facilitating change [5]. MI requires a nuanced connection with the patient and evolves with hands-on experience where practitioners learn that maintaining a connection requires revisiting engagement techniques multiple times within a session, as conversations about VH can ebb and flow. Each patient interaction is a learning opportunity, providing invaluable insights that refine the practitioner's approach and enhance their ability to tailor conversations to individual concerns [72]. If patient engagement is lost, the practitioner is best advised to take a step back and attempt to re-engage the patient [15]. Becoming proficient in MI techniques involves more than just learning the methods; it involves integrating these skills into practice naturally and effectively.

7.9 Applying Motivational Interviewing to Practice

Incorporating MI into daily practice is often one of the most challenging steps for general practitioners [73]. Even though MI is a valuable tool, it is only as good as the practitioner who uses it. To introduce the skill in many settings, preclinical and clinical educators have been tailoring MI simulations to train healthcare workers to respond to many scenarios appropriately. What often stays consistent across these simulations are the core skills of MI and whether the practitioner adequately understands them. Multiple studies have suggested that MI training has commonly improved interview competency with students and professionals, leading to behavioral changes in patients exposed to those trained in it [74–76].

For MI to continue to be effective, clinicians need to maintain their skills. In their 2014 meta-analysis, Schwalbe et al. found that for maintaining MI skills among trainees, especially in the context of treating substance use disorders, it is beneficial to have three to four feedback or coaching sessions over 6 months [77]. Enhanced MI Skills Code (MISC) scores have demonstrated improvements in MI skills, leading to better patient results. These improvements include better empathy, adherence to MI spirit, more effective reflective listening, reduced use of closed-ended questions, and advising without permission, as reported by Magill et al. in their 2010 study [78].

One of the critical steps is incorporating OARS techniques. During the actual session, MI employs various skills to address VH, explicitly utilizing the OARS technique: open questions to delve into the patient's vaccine-related concerns, affirmation to reinforce their confidence in health decision-making, reflective listening for a deeper understanding of their attitudes toward vaccines, and the elicit–share–elicit method for offering advice in a structured manner. Through these approaches, MI focuses on affirming the patient's priorities and fostering an open information exchange. Subsequently, pertinent vaccine information is shared, addressing any specific concerns they may have.

Here is an example of an OARS-focus session for VH:

1. *Open questions:* What are your concerns about the MMR vaccine?
2. *Affirmation:* The health and safety of your children are your top priority, and you are concerned about the side effects of vaccines.
3. *Reflective listening:* It is my understanding that you have researched the MMR vaccine and are worried about the relationships between vaccines and autism.
4. *Elicit–share–elicit:* Would you be open to me providing the experience I have learned about vaccines and their relationship to autism? [Share your experience] What are some questions you may have about the information I have shared?

If a patient is positioned within the hesitant portion of the VH spectrum, pinpointing their specific concerns through the framework of the 5 Cs—confidence, complacency, convenience, calculation, and collective responsibility—provides a valuable starting point for practitioners [49]. The practitioner can tailor their approach more effectively by understanding which factors predominantly influence the patient's hesitancy. This tailored approach allows the practitioner to utilize the OARS technique to engage the patient in a meaningful dialogue about their concerns [5]. Identifying concerns based on the 5 Cs facilitates a focused conversation, where the practitioner can address specific misunderstandings or fears, building trust and openness. Through the application of OARS, the practitioner encourages the patient to express their views and feelings in a nonjudgmental environment, enhancing the likelihood of progressing toward acceptance [5]. This strategic engagement acknowledges the patient's autonomy and gently guides them toward reconsidering their stance on vaccination, making it a crucial step for those in the hesitant space.

7.9.1 Motivational Interviewing Resources

A wealth of resources, such as expert-authored books and practical workbooks, play an indispensable role in supporting the practical application of MI. These tools deepen understanding and provide practical avenues for patients and professionals to refine their MI skills, fostering a more informed and empowered approach to healthcare decisions.

Printed Materials and Workbooks For those preferring tangible resources, printed materials and workbooks play a pivotal role in reinforcing the concepts of MI. Books authored by experts in the field, such as "MI: Helping People Change" by William R. Miller and Stephen Rollnick, serve as comprehensive guides for those seeking more profound insights into the methodology [5]. Workbooks incorporating exercises and reflection prompts, such as "Building Motivational Interviewing Skills: A Practitioner Workbook" by David B. Rosengren, offer practical applications to reinforce learning outside clinical settings [22].

Empowering patients with readily accessible resources fosters self-efficacy and reinforces the principles learned through clinical encounters. By offering a spectrum of resources—from online modules to community workshops—patients are equipped with the tools necessary to embrace and sustain behavioral changes, ultimately creating a collaborative and effective healthcare experience.

VH, at its core, is multi-faceted and, for many people, is deep-rooted in perceptions, often influenced by cultural, religious, or historical contexts. This complex web of beliefs takes time to resolve with MI. Furthermore, tools available to the public such as social media have been found to have a substantial relationship in the prevalence of doubts about vaccine safety that can increase as greater online organizations and foreign disinformation appear [79]. Even before the COVID-19 pandemic, opinions about vaccines were reported to become more polarized throughout the 2010s [79]. This trend has continued during the pandemic, where reliance on social media posts has been associated with higher levels of VH in both the public and healthcare workers [80]. While social media is a threat to worsening levels of VH, it may also play a part in the solution. A systematic review by Li et al. found that using social media to deploy behavioral change theory-based countermeasures, such as informational posts or interactive websites, increased vaccine confidence and vaccine uptake [81]. This study also saw positive results with the use of online dialogue-based groups where MI techniques can be used to encourage discussion [81]. While the modern world faces a growing amount of VH, there are also many ways to combat this hesitancy using MI or related behavioral change-based techniques both in person and online.

7.10 Conclusion

VH remains a significant barrier to achieving widespread immunization and preventing the resurgence of vaccine-preventable diseases. VH exists on a spectrum, ranging from complete refusal to cautious acceptance, with various psychological, social, and cultural factors influencing individuals' decisions. Mistrust in healthcare systems, misinformation, concerns about vaccine safety, and personal beliefs all contribute to VH, making it a complex and persistent challenge for public health.

MI has emerged as an effective approach to addressing VH by fostering open, non-confrontational conversations that respect patient autonomy. Unlike traditional methods of persuasion, which may lead to resistance or disengagement, MI seeks to understand the root causes of VH and tailor discussions accordingly. The MI framework enables healthcare providers to identify where a patient falls on the VH continuum and adapt their approach using key principles: expressing empathy, developing discrepancy, rolling with resistance, and supporting self-efficacy.

Developed as a collaborative and empathetic approach, MI prioritizes active listening, reflective questioning, and patient autonomy to encourage individuals to make informed health decisions. The technique is structured around four key principles: expressing empathy, developing discrepancy, rolling with resistance, and supporting self-efficacy. Unlike traditional persuasive methods that may provoke resistance, MI engages individuals in a nonconfrontational dialogue that aligns with their values and motivations. Through strategic questioning and affirmations, healthcare providers can guide patients toward recognizing inconsistencies between their concerns and their health goals, ultimately fostering a sense of ownership over their decision-making process.

A critical application of MI is in addressing VH, a multifaceted issue influenced by social, psychological, and cultural factors. VH exists along a spectrum, ranging from full vaccine acceptance to outright vaccine refusal. Individuals at the most resistant end—vaccine deniers—reject all immunizations, often due to deeply entrenched beliefs and mistrust in medical institutions. Vaccine refusers may be skeptical but are more open to reconsidering their stance under certain conditions. The hesitant middle includes those who delay vaccination due to concerns about safety, efficacy, or necessity, while cautious acceptors generally follow recommended schedules but may have lingering doubts. Understanding where a patient falls on this spectrum allows healthcare providers to tailor MI strategies accordingly, ensuring that interventions are appropriately targeted to the patient's level of readiness for change.

One of the most powerful aspects of MI in combating VH is its ability to counter misinformation in a way that does not alienate patients. Many hesitant individuals base their concerns on anecdotal experiences, social influences, or cognitive biases rather than scientific evidence. MI allows providers to gently challenge these beliefs by guiding patients toward reconciling their concerns with their health goals. By asking open-ended questions, actively listening, and reinforcing a patient's own motivations for protecting their health, MI fosters trust and increases vaccine acceptance.

Research has demonstrated that MI can be highly effective in vaccine-related discussions, particularly in pediatric and primary care settings. Studies show that even brief MI interventions can significantly improve vaccine uptake, especially when healthcare providers integrate MI techniques into routine conversations. Parents hesitant about childhood vaccines, for example, are more likely to consider immunization schedules when they feel heard, understood, and guided rather than coerced. Similarly, adults hesitant about new vaccines, such as those developed for COVID-19 or HPV, may be more open to vaccination after engaging in an MI-based discussion that respects their concerns and provides clear, evidence-based information.

The ongoing challenge of VH requires a multifaceted approach, and MI plays a critical role in bridging the gap between hesitancy and acceptance. As vaccine misinformation proliferates online and skepticism toward public health institutions persists, MI offers a sustainable and scalable solution for healthcare professionals to engage with hesitant individuals effectively. Training healthcare providers in MI techniques will be essential in equipping them with the skills necessary to navigate difficult conversations, address specific patient concerns, and promote vaccine confidence.

Ultimately, MI is not just a tool for persuasion—it is a method for fostering long-term trust and encouraging patients to make informed health decisions. By addressing the psychological and social dimensions of VH with empathy and collaboration, MI enhances the effectiveness of vaccine promotion efforts and contributes to improved public health outcomes. Future research should focus on refining MI-based interventions for specific populations, integrating MI into digital health communication strategies, and assessing the long-term impact of MI on vaccine acceptance across different communities.

References

1. Josephson H, Carlbring P, Forsberg L, Rosendahl I. People with gambling disorder and risky alcohol habits benefit more from motivational interviewing than from cognitive behavioral group therapy. PeerJ. 2016;4:e1899. https://doi.org/10.7717/peerj.1899.
2. Hettema J, Steele J, Miller WR. Motivational interviewing. Annu Rev Clin Psychol. 2005;1(1):91–111. https://doi.org/10.1146/annurev.clinpsy.1.102803.143833.
3. Louwagie GMC, Okuyemi KS, Ayo-Yusuf OA. Efficacy of brief motivational interviewing on smoking cessation at tuberculosis clinics in Tshwane, South Africa: a randomized controlled trial. Addiction. 2014;109(11):1942–52. https://doi.org/10.1111/add.12671.

4. Taheri F, Nasiri A, Namdari S, Salmani F. Effect of motivational interviewing on treatment adherence and SELF-EFFICACY of adolescents with asthma: a randomized controlled trial. Nurs Open. 2023;10(7):4373–83. https://doi.org/10.1002/nop2.1679.
5. Miller W, Rollnick S. Motivational interviewing fourth edition helping people change and grow. 4th ed. Guilford Press; 2023.
6. COVID vaccine confidence requires radical transparency. Nature. 2020;586(7827):8–8. https://doi.org/10.1038/d41586-020-02738-y.
7. Gagneur A, Lemaître T, Gosselin V, et al. A postpartum vaccination promotion intervention using motivational interviewing techniques improves short-term vaccine coverage: PromoVac study. BMC Public Health. 2018;18(1):811. https://doi.org/10.1186/s12889-018-5724-y.
8. Zolezzi M, Paravattil B, El-Gaili T. Using motivational interviewing techniques to inform decision-making for COVID-19 vaccination. Int J Clin Pharm. 2021;43(6):1728–34. https://doi.org/10.1007/s11096-021-01334-y.
9. Dubé E, Laberge C, Guay M, Bramadat P, Roy R, Bettinger J. Vaccine hesitancy: an overview. Hum Vaccin Immunother. 2013;9(8):1763–73. https://doi.org/10.4161/hv.24657.
10. Borga LG, Clark AE, D'Ambrosio C, Lepinteur A. Characteristics associated with COVID-19 vaccine hesitancy. Sci Rep. 2022;12(1):12435. https://doi.org/10.1038/s41598-022-16572-x.
11. Opel DJ, Salmon DA, Marcuse EK. Building trust to achieve confidence in COVID-19 vaccines. JAMA Netw Open. 2020;3(10):e2025672. https://doi.org/10.1001/jamanetworkopen.2020.25672.
12. Boness CL, Nelson M, Douaihy AB. Motivational interviewing strategies for addressing COVID-19 vaccine hesitancy. J Am Board Fam Med. 2022;35(2):420–6. https://doi.org/10.3122/jabfm.2022.02.210327.
13. Breckenridge LA, Burns D, Nye C. The use of motivational interviewing to overcome COVID-19 vaccine hesitancy in primary care settings. Public Health Nurs. 2022;39(3):618–23. https://doi.org/10.1111/phn.13003.
14. Miller WR. The evolution of motivational interviewing. Behav Cogn Psychother. 2023;51:616–32. https://doi.org/10.1017/S1352465822000431.
15. Bischof G, Bischof A, Rumpf HJ. Motivational interviewing: an evidence-based approach for use in medical practice. Dtsch Arztebl Int. 2021;118(7):109–15. https://doi.org/10.3238/arztebl.m2021.0014.
16. Treasure J. Motivational interviewing. Adv Psychiatr Treat. 2004;10(5):331–7. https://doi.org/10.1192/apt.10.5.331.
17. Frost H, Campbell P, Maxwell M, et al. Effectiveness of motivational interviewing on adult behaviour change in health and social care settings: a systematic review of reviews. PLoS One. 2018;13(10):e0204890. https://doi.org/10.1371/journal.pone.0204890.
18. Miller WR, Rose GS. Motivational interviewing and decisional balance: contrasting responses to client ambivalence. Behav Cogn Psychother. 2015;43(2):129–41. https://doi.org/10.1017/S1352465813000878.
19. Lim D, Schoo A, Lawn S, Litt J. Embedding and sustaining motivational interviewing in clinical environments: a concurrent iterative mixed methods study. BMC Med Educ. 2019;19(1):164. https://doi.org/10.1186/s12909-019-1606-y.
20. Hedegaard U, Kjeldsen LJ, Pottegård A, et al. Improving medication adherence in patients with hypertension: a randomized trial. Am J Med. 2015;128(12):1351–61. https://doi.org/10.1016/j.amjmed.2015.08.011.
21. Miller WR, Rollnick S. Motivational interviewing: preparing people to change addictive behavior. New York: Guilford Press; 1991, 1991. Pp. xvii + 348. £24.95 hardback, £11.50 paper. ISBN 0–89862–566–1 – Bennett – 1992 – Journal of Community & Applied Social Psychology – Wiley Online Library. Accessed 20 Oct 2023. https://onlinelibrary-wiley-com.proxy.rvu.edu/doi/abs/10.1002/casp.2450020410.
22. Rosengren DB. Building motivational interviewing skills: a practitioner workbook. 1st ed. Guilford Press; 2012.

23. CDC. Measles Cases and Outbreaks. Centers for Disease Control and Prevention. September 12, 2023. Accessed 13 Sept 2023. https://www.cdc.gov/measles/cases-outbreaks.html.
24. Christie D, Channon S. The potential for motivational interviewing to improve outcomes in the management of diabetes and obesity in paediatric and adult populations: a clinical review. Diabetes Obes Metab. 2013;16:381. https://doi.org/10.1111/dom.12195.
25. Rollnick S, Miller WR, Butler C, Aloia MS. Motivational interviewing in health care: helping patients change behavior. Am J Pharm Educ. 2008; https://doi.org/10.1080/15412550802093108.
26. Guo B, Aveyard P, Fielding A, Sutton S. Do the Transtheoretical Model processes of change, decisional balance and temptation predict stage movement? Evidence from smoking cessation in adolescents. Addiction. 2009;104(5):828–38. https://doi.org/10.1111/j.1360-0443.2009.02519.x.
27. Harrell PT, Trenz RC, Scherer M, Martins SS, Latimer WW. A latent class approach to treatment readiness corresponds to a transtheoretical ("Stages of Change") model. J Subst Abus Treat. 2013;45(3):249–56. https://doi.org/10.1016/j.jsat.2013.04.004.
28. Petrocelli JV. Processes and stages of change: counseling with the transtheoretical model of change. J Couns Dev. 2002;80(1):22–30. https://doi.org/10.1002/j.1556-6678.2002.tb00162.x.
29. Time for a change: putting the Transtheoretical (Stages of Change) Model to rest. Addiction. 2005;100(8):1036–9. https://doi.org/10.1111/j.1360-0443.2005.01139.x.
30. Miller WR, Rollnick S. Motivational interviewing: preparing people for change. 2nd ed. Guilford Press; 2002.
31. Miller WR, Rose GS. Toward a theory of motivational interviewing. Am Psychol. 2009;64(6):527–37. https://doi.org/10.1037/a0016830.
32. Ingersoll K. Substance use disorders: motivational interviewing. UpToDate. Published online February 20, 2024. https://www-uptodate-com.proxy.rvu.edu/contents/substance-use-disorders-motivational-interviewing?search=Substance%20use%20disorders%3A%20Motivational%20interviewing&source=search_result&selectedTitle=1%7E150&usage_type=default&display_rank=1.
33. Lundahl BW, Kunz C, Brownell C, Tollefson D, Burke BL. A meta-analysis of motivational interviewing: twenty-five years of empirical studies. Res Soc Work Pract. 2010;20(2):137–60. https://doi.org/10.1177/1049731509347850.
34. Ghaderi A, Rosendahl I, Bohman B. Integrating motivational interviewing with cognitive behavioural therapy for anxiety disorders, depression and co-morbid unhealthy lifestyle behaviours: a randomised controlled pilot trial. Behav Cogn Psychother. 2022;50(1):74–88. https://doi.org/10.1017/S1352465821000345.
35. Westra H. Managing resistance in cognitive behavioural therapy: the application of motivational interviewing in mixed anxiety and depression. Cogn Behav Ther. 2004;33(4):161–75. https://doi.org/10.1080/16506070410026426.
36. Gillam DG, Yusuf H. Brief motivational interviewing in dental practice. Dentistry Journal. 2019;7(2):51. https://doi.org/10.3390/dj7020051.
37. VanBuskirk KA, Wetherell JL. Motivational interviewing with primary care populations: a systematic review and meta-analysis. J Behav Med. 2014;37(4):768–80. https://doi.org/10.1007/s10865-013-9527-4.
38. Del Giudice MJ, Kutinsky J. Applying motivational interviewing to the treatment of sexual compulsivity and addiction. Sex Addict Compuls. 2007;14(4):303–19. https://doi.org/10.1080/10720160701710634.
39. Burke BL, Arkowitz H, Menchola M. The efficacy of motivational interviewing: a meta-analysis of controlled clinical trials. J Consult Clin Psychol. 2003;71(5):843–61. https://doi.org/10.1037/0022-006X.71.5.843.
40. Lundahl B, Burke BL. The effectiveness and applicability of motivational interviewing: a practice-friendly review of four meta-analyses. J Clin Psychol. 2009;65(11):1232–45. https://doi.org/10.1002/jclp.20638.

41. Rubak S, Sandbæk A, Lauritzen T, Christensen B. Motivational interviewing: a systematic review and meta-analysis. Br J Gen Pract. 2005;55(513):305–12.
42. Pace BT, Dembe A, Soma CS, Baldwin SA, Atkins DC, Imel ZE. A multivariate meta-analysis of motivational interviewing process and outcome. Psychol Addict Behav. 2017;31(5):524–33. https://doi.org/10.1037/adb0000280.
43. Qiqi N, Hangting L, Jia W, Jiaoni S, Xinrui W, Guijuan H. A meta-analysis of the effect of motivational interviewing on depression, anxiety, and quality of life in stroke patients. J Neurosci Nurs. 2021;53(6):244–50. https://doi.org/10.1097/JNN.0000000000000617.
44. Magill M, Apodaca TR, Borsari B, et al. A meta-analysis of motivational interviewing process: technical, relational, and conditional process models of change. J Consult Clin Psychol. 2018;86(2):140–57. https://doi.org/10.1037/ccp0000250.
45. Cole JW, Chen AMH, McGuire K, Berman S, Gardner J, Teegala Y. Motivational interviewing and vaccine acceptance in children: the MOTIVE study. Vaccine. 2022;40(12):1846–54. https://doi.org/10.1016/j.vaccine.2022.01.058.
46. MacDonald N. Vaccine hesitancy: definition, scope and determinants. Vaccine. 33:4161. https://doi.org/10.1016/j.vaccine.2015.04.036.
47. Gill C. Vaccine hesitancy: how did we get here and what do we do now? SPH. Published online March 1, 2022. https://www.bu.edu/sph/news/articles/2022/covid-19-vaccine-hesitancy-how-did-we-get-here-and-what-do-we-do-now/
48. MacDonald N. Fake news and science denier attacks on vaccines. What can you do? Can Commun Dis Rep. Published online November 5, 2020. https://doi.org/10.14745/ccdr.v46i1112a11.
49. Betsch C, Schmid P, Heinemeier D, Korn L, Holtmann C, Böhm R. Beyond confidence: development of a measure assessing the 5C psychological antecedents of vaccination. PLoS One. 2018;13(12):e0208601. https://doi.org/10.1371/journal.pone.0208601.
50. Plitch-Leob R, Silver D, Kim Y, Norris H, McNeil E. Determinants of the COVID-19 vaccine hesitancy spectrum. PLoS One. Published online June 1, 2022. https://doi.org/10.1371/journal.pone.0267734.
51. Cushman F. Rationalization is rational. Behav Brain Sci. 2019;43:e28. https://doi.org/10.1017/S0140525X19001730.
52. Rancher C, Moreland A, Smith D. Using the 5C model to understand COVID-19 vaccine hesitancy across a National and South Carolina sample. J Psychiatr Res. 160:180. https://doi.org/10.1016/j.jpsychires.2023.02.018.
53. Rodriguez VJ, Kozlova S, LaBarrie DL, Liu Q. Parental anxiety and pediatric vaccine refusal in a US national sample of parents. Vaccine. 2023;41(48):7072–5. https://doi.org/10.1016/j.vaccine.2023.10.015.
54. Davis TC, Vanchiere JA, Sewell MR, Davis AB, Wolf MS, Arnold CL. Influenza and COVID-19 vaccine concerns and uptake among patients cared for in a safety-net health system. J Prim Care Community Health. 2022;13:21501319221136361. https://doi.org/10.1177/21501319221136361.
55. Brown K, Kroll J. Factors underlying parental decisions about combination childhood vaccinations including MMR: a systematic review. Vaccine. 28:4235. https://doi.org/10.1016/j.vaccine.2010.04.052.
56. Santoro C. Vaccine hesitancy fuels global health crisis amidst multidisease outbreaks. AJMC. Published online August 8, 2024. https://www.ajmc.com/view/vaccine-hesitancy-fuels-global-health-crisis-amidst-multi-disease-outbreaks.
57. Almadani O, Alshammari T. Vaccine adverse event reporting system (VAERS): evaluation of 31 years of reports and pandemics' impact. Saudi Pharm J. Published online October 2022. https://doi.org/10.1016/j.jsps.2022.10.001
58. Jamieson K, Johnson K, Cappola A. Misinformation and the vaccine adverse event reporting system. JAMA. 331:1005. https://doi.org/10.1001/jama.2024.1757.
59. CDC. Adult vaccination coverage and intent. COVIDVaxView. Published online 2024. https://www.cdc.gov/covidvaxview/weekly-dashboard/adult-vaccination-coverage.html.

60. Feemster KA, Szipszky C. Resurgence of measles in the United States: how did we get here? Curr Opin Pediatr. 2020;32(1):139–44. https://doi.org/10.1097/MOP.0000000000000845.
61. Brouwer AF, Delinger RL, Eisenberg MC, et al. HPV vaccination has not increased sexual activity or accelerated sexual debut in a college-aged cohort of men and women. BMC Public Health. 2019;19(1):821. https://doi.org/10.1186/s12889-019-7134-1.
62. Kata A. Anti-vaccine activists, Web 2.0, and the postmodern paradigm – an overview of tactics and tropes used online by the anti-vaccination movement. Vaccine. Published online 2012. https://doi.org/10.1016/j.vaccine.2011.11.112.
63. Cunningham-Erves J, Hull PC, Wilkins CH, et al. Healthcare providers' practice protocols, strategies, and needed tools to address parental HPV vaccine hesitancy: an exploratory study. Hum Vaccin Immunother. 18(6):2136862. https://doi.org/10.1080/21645515.2022.2136862.
64. Kolobova I, Nyaku MK, Karakusevic A, Bridge D, Fotheringham I, O'Brien M. Burden of vaccine-preventable diseases among at-risk adult populations in the US. Hum Vaccin Immunother. 2022;18(5):2054602. https://doi.org/10.1080/21645515.2022.2054602.
65. Galagali PM, Kinikar AA, Kumar VS. Vaccine hesitancy: obstacles and challenges. Curr Pediatr Rep. 2022;10(4):241–8. https://doi.org/10.1007/s40124-022-00278-9.
66. Hofstetter AM, Opel DJ, Stockwell MS, et al. Influenza-related knowledge, beliefs, and experiences among caregivers of hospitalized children. Hosp Pediatr. 2021;11(8):815–32. https://doi.org/10.1542/hpeds.2020-003459.
67. Gagneur A. Motivational interviewing: a powerful tool to address vaccine hesitancy. Can Commun Dis Rep. 2020;46(4):93–7. https://doi.org/10.14745/ccdr.v46i04a06.
68. Lemaitre T, Carrier N, Farrands A, Gosselin V, Petit G, Gagneur A. Impact of a vaccination promotion intervention using motivational interview techniques on long-term vaccine coverage: the PromoVac strategy. Hum Vaccin Immunother. 2019;15(3):732–9. https://doi.org/10.1080/21645515.2018.1549451.
69. Gagneur A, Battista M, Boucher F. Promoting vaccination in maternity wards – motivational interview technique reduces hesitancy and enhances intention to vaccinate, results from a multicentre non-controlled pre- and post-intervention RCT-nested study, Quebec, March 2014 to February 2015. Euro Surveill. Published online 2019. https://doi.org/10.2807/1560-7917.ES.2019.24.36.1800641.
70. Dempsey AF, Pyrznawoski J, Lockhart S, et al. Effect of a health care professional communication training intervention on adolescent human papillomavirus vaccination. JAMA Pediatr. 2018;172(5):e180016. https://doi.org/10.1001/jamapediatrics.2018.0016.
71. Vaccine hesitancy: contemporary issues and historical background – PMC. Accessed 15 Feb 2024. https://www.ncbi.nlm.nih.gov/pmc/articles/PMC9612044/.
72. Wallace L. Learning motivational interviewing: a thematic analysis exploring health professionals' training experiences. Thesis. Queen Margaret University; 2011. Accessed 15 Feb 2024. https://eresearch.qmu.ac.uk/handle/20.500.12289/7734.
73. Boom SM, Oberink R, Zonneveld AJE, van Dijk N, Visser MRM. Implementation of motivational interviewing in the general practice setting: a qualitative study. BMC Prim Care. 2022;23:21. https://doi.org/10.1186/s12875-022-01623-z.
74. Edwards EJ, Arora B, Green P, Bannatyne AJ, Nielson T. Teaching brief motivational interviewing to medical students using a pedagogical framework. Patient Educ Couns. 2022;105(7):2315–9. https://doi.org/10.1016/j.pec.2022.01.012.
75. Barwick MA, Bennett LM, Johnson SN, McGowan J, Moore JE. Training health and mental health professionals in motivational interviewing: a systematic review. Child Youth Serv Rev. 2012;34(9):1786–95. https://doi.org/10.1016/j.childyouth.2012.05.012.
76. Martino S, Haeseler F, Belitsky R, Pantalon M, Fortin AH IV. Teaching brief motivational interviewing to year three medical students. Med Educ. 2007;41(2):160–7. https://doi.org/10.1111/j.1365-2929.2006.02673.x.
77. Schwalbe CS, Oh HY, Zweben A. Sustaining motivational interviewing: a meta-analysis of training studies. Addiction. 2014;109(8):1287–94. https://doi.org/10.1111/add.12558.

78. Magill M, Mastroleo NR, Apodaca TR, Barnett NP, Colby SM, Monti PM. Motivational interviewing with significant other participation: assessing therapeutic alliance and patient satisfaction and engagement. J Subst Abus Treat. 2010;39(4):391–8. https://doi.org/10.1016/j.jsat.2010.07.006.
79. Piedrahita-Valdés H, Piedrahita-Castillo D, Bermejo-Higuera J, et al. Vaccine hesitancy on social media: sentiment analysis from June 2011 to April 2019. Vaccine. 2021;9(1):28. https://doi.org/10.3390/vaccines9010028.
80. Rodrigues F, Ziade N, Jatuworapruk K, Caballero-Uribe CV, Khursheed T, Gupta L. The impact of social media on vaccination: a narrative review. J Korean Med Sci. 2023;38(40):e326. https://doi.org/10.3346/jkms.2023.38.e326.
81. Li L, Wood CE, Kostkova P. Vaccine hesitancy and behavior change theory-based social media interventions: a systematic review. Transl Behav Med. 2022;12(2):243–72. https://doi.org/10.1093/tbm/ibab148.

Chapter 8
Community-Based Vaccine Education and Initiatives

Andrea Levin, Raisa Khan, Patricia Milanes, Sheena Pubien, Emmanuela Beliard, and Laci Rae-Pitter

8.1 Considering Community Needs in Vaccine Education and Initiatives

8.1.1 Health Needs

Vaccines are highly effective at preventing infectious diseases, demonstrating their potential to eradicate and/or diminish the prevalence of deadly or disabling infections such as smallpox and measles [1]. Therefore, adherence to vaccination guidelines is crucial for community well-being, with lower rates of vaccination posing threats to immunity and causing the resurgence of vaccine-preventable diseases. However, vaccination rates exhibit significant variability across communities and demographics, highlighting the need to comprehend and address the unique needs of specific populations.

Every community has its own distinct set of health needs and challenges that impede proper vaccination. For instance, migrant communities often have lower vaccination rates, which can partially be attributed to factors such as differing vaccination schedules compared to their country of origin, incomplete medical and vaccination records, and uncertainty regarding their vaccination status [1]. Moreover,

A. Levin (✉)
Nova Southeastern University, Barry and Judy Silverman College of Pharmacy, Fort Lauderdale, FL, USA
e-mail: afass@nova.edu

R. Khan · P. Milanes · S. Pubien · L. Rae-Pitter
Nova Southeastern University, Dr. Kiran C. Patel College of Allopathic Medicine, Fort Lauderdale, FL, USA

E. Beliard
New York Institute of Technology College of Osteopathic Medicine-Arkansas, Jonesboro, AR, USA

A. J. Chase et al. (eds.), *Vaccine Hesitancy Curriculum*,
https://doi.org/10.1007/978-3-031-88668-3_8

inadequately trained healthcare professionals may inadvertently overlook catch-up vaccination opportunities, further exacerbated by language barriers that impede effective communication [2].

Cultural perspectives also exert a profound influence, with certain communities harboring perceptions of vaccines as either risky or lacking benefits. For instance, Romanian and Romanian Roma populations consider contracting measles as a "rite of passage" for children or believe the vaccines were not effective [1, 3]. This once again highlights the different concerns each community has regarding vaccinations, and the presence of community advocates and culturally sensitive healthcare providers has been shown to increase vaccination rates, showing the importance of culturally competent engagement.

Parental concerns further shape vaccination rates, with fears of severe side effects and doubts about vaccine efficacy acting as significant barriers. One survey about the influenza vaccine showed that parents may not choose to vaccinate due to the belief that the vaccine is ineffective and the lack of perceived risk of the influenza virus [4]. Many parents have expressed their reluctance toward vaccinating their children with the HPV vaccine, interpreting immunization against a sexually transmitted infection as permissive of sexual promiscuity. Clinicians should take a comprehensive pediatric social history, especially to identify children who are homeschooled. In the United States, low immunization rates are seen in homeschooled pediatric populations, given a lack of school mandates for vaccination and varying state laws on immunization requirements for homeschooled children [5, 6]. Some parents have opted to homeschool their children for the express purpose of avoiding educational system vaccine mandates, and outbreaks of vaccine-preventable illness have been associated with communities in which homeschooling is common. Understanding parents' specific concerns and addressing apprehensions through education and goal-oriented communication may help diminish vaccine hesitancy. Healthcare providers should exercise judgment and use open-ended questioning to assess where parents/patients stand and the values that guide their decisions, especially when such conversations can be incredibly sensitive [7].

Take the following example scenario of discussing the HPV vaccine with a parent who is hesitant to consent for their child to receive it. Healthcare providers may begin by asking, "Would you be willing to share your thoughts regarding the HPV vaccine?" or "What do you know or what have you heard about the HPV vaccine?" Clinicians may encounter the reasoning that a parent considers their child/the recommended age for vaccination (11–12 years) to be too young to engage in sexual activity/have exposure to HPV. Parents should be made aware that the vaccine is most effective in preventing HPV-associated cancers when administered prior to exposure. Parents may also be more receptive if informed HPV transmission is still possible through saliva/mouth-to-mouth contact, behavior they may consider to be more acceptable for a preteen. Clinicians should gauge parents' openness to discuss the possibility that their child might currently, if not soon, engage in sexual activity. It is estimated that over half of teens in the United States have been sexually active before the age of 18. This subject is a difficult one to broach, as not all parents are willing to believe that their children are engaging in sexual activity as minors. Many parents believe that simply talking about sex with their children may inherently signal permission of the act and may decline HPV vaccines because they may view it as a "green light" for sexual activity. Others may not feel that the time-sensitivity of HPV vaccine administration is not relevant to their child—the response to being informed about national statistics of teens who are sexually active as minors may very well be: "Not my kid." Many parents do not want to consider the possibility that their children may not be forthcoming with their parents about whether they are sexually active. Moreover, not only do parents typically have expectations of their children's behavior, but it is also likely that parents have expectations of their children's future partners. It is important to acknowledge the stigma of having a sexually transmitted infection, its association with sexual promiscuity, and that many parents do not want to believe that their child would engage in sexual activity with someone whom parents believe to be/have been sexually promiscuous. Clinicians may additionally encounter parents whose beliefs, religious or otherwise, are that their child is to remain abstinent until marriage, therefore not requiring the HPV vaccine before then. Parents may still struggle to accept that their child's future spouse could expose them to HPV, but they may be more amenable to vaccinating their child when this possibility is brought to their attention. This scenario highlights that there may be a host of psychosocial factors influencing a parent's decision, and clinicians should take care to identify and address concerns with sensitivity.

It is important to highlight that patients' health status can delineate other demographics to consider in education and immunization initiatives. Patients with specific medical conditions may have unique vaccination needs—e.g., additional pneumococcal vaccine doses may be indicated for individuals with risk conditions, including but not limited to diabetes mellitus, chronic liver disease, sickle cell disease, and other immunocompromising conditions [8]. The prevalence of certain health conditions in some demographics (and any resulting unique vaccination needs) must be discussed in conjunction with demographic-specific structural barriers to care/vaccination. For example, the incidence of sickle cell disease is higher in African American populations relative to other demographics, and lower vaccination rates have been seen in this same community. Clinicians must understand that this combination of health disparities and socioeconomic factors can lead to those patient populations most needing vaccination having the most barriers to being vaccinated. Individuals living with disabilities are a population that experiences often unacknowledged health inequities, including lower vaccination rates. Trauma in healthcare settings (including both personal and historic provider judgment and/or discrimination), uncertainty about how certain vaccines may interact with health conditions, and barriers to physical access have all been cited as contributors to vaccine hesitancy for people living with disabilities.

Access to healthcare is pivotal in increasing vaccination rates, emphasizing the necessity of expanding healthcare accessibility and extending vaccination services to community settings. Tailored public health initiatives targeting the specific concerns and public nuances of diverse communities are essential for fostering trust and compliance with vaccination recommendations and ultimately contribute to the well-being of the public on a broad scale.

8.1.2 Demographic-Specific Historical Barriers

Vaccination can mitigate the transmission of infectious diseases while also diminishing mortality and morbidity yet vaccination rates in ethnic minorities, socially and economically marginalized populations, and rural communities have continued to remain low [9]. Historically, certain factors have been identified that have increased vaccine hesitancy among certain demographics. Some bases of vaccine hesitancy among certain demographics may be in part due to medical mistrust. According to the World Health Organization (WHO) Strategic Advisory Group of Experts on Immunization (SAGE), vaccine hesitancy is defined as follows: "Vaccine hesitancy refers to delay in acceptance or refusal of vaccines despite availability of vaccination services" [10]. Recognition of these historical barriers to vaccine uptake permits healthcare providers to address disparities in vaccine uptake and tailor interventions to fit the needs of their community demographic.

As previously discussed, medical mistrust may serve as a primary catalyst for vaccine hesitancy in specific populations. Numerous historical events of unethical medical practices, such as the Tuskegee Syphilis experiment, forced sterilization and the general exclusion of minorities from clinical trials have all garnered mistrust among patients, particularly among Black, Hispanic, and Indigenous communities [11, 12]. Medical mistrust has been implicated as an attitudinal barrier to vaccine uptake among ethnic minorities, socially and economically marginalized populations, and rural communities [9]. There have also been disproven concerns about vaccine safety as seen with HPV vaccines and aluminum in vaccines increasing the risk of autoimmune disorders, which ha lead to the spread of misinformation and a decrease in vaccine uptake [13]. In addition, the 1998 dissemination of the false claim of the potential linkage of MMR (measles, mumps, rubella) vaccination to autism has had profound consequences in causing widespread mistrust in medical providers and skepticism in vaccines [14]. Sluggish mobilization of the larger medical community and structural violence embedded in policy during the HIV/AIDS epidemic in the 1980s has had a profound effect on how LGBTQ+ communities interact with the healthcare system [15]. Populations at the intersection of race, gender identity, and sexual orientation also experience health and vaccination disparities, with low immunization rates seen among Black LGBT individuals, particularly those who identify as women [16]. This disparity is particularly deserving of our attention, especially considering that members of the LGBTQ+ community are at increased risk for contracting some vaccine-preventable conditions, such as Hepatitis B. For groups that may already be marginalized and underrepresented in the healthcare community, ingroup–outgroup biases may reinforce a sense of mistrust and division [17, 18]. As a result, these aforementioned events have significantly weakened public trust in the healthcare system further leading to the hindrance of efforts to promote vaccination, especially in populations particularly vulnerable to vaccine-preventable diseases.

Ultimately, vaccination plays a crucial role in protecting individuals and communities from the spread of infectious diseases. However, there are several historical barriers that prevent certain demographics from opting to receive immunizations. Identification of historical barriers will allow healthcare providers to recognize the root causes of medical mistrust and vaccine hesitancy. Also, remaining cognizant of these barriers will allow healthcare providers to make more informed decisions when designing vaccination programs to better fit the demographic(s) in need and ensuring education endeavors are community-appropriate, employing demographic-specific strategies for effective communication [19, 20]. Furthermore, making efforts to build trust with their patients while addressing misconceptions about vaccines may help increase vaccine uptake in vulnerable populations [21].

8.1.3 Accessibility Needs

Vaccination stands as the most effective method in mitigating the transmission of infectious diseases while also diminishing mortality and morbidity [22]. The Centers for Disease Control and Prevention (CDC) estimates that among U.S. adults, there are approximately 40,000 cases and 4000 deaths associated with pneumococcal disease; in addition, there are between 3000 and 49,000 deaths due to seasonal influenza annually [23]. However, low vaccination rates continue to persist within specific demographics such as ethnic minorities, socially and economically marginalized populations, and rural communities due to challenges affecting vaccine access [24]. Vaccine access or convenience is the degree to which physical, geographical, and language proficiency factors influence vaccine compliance and uptake [25, 26]. Identification of barriers to vaccine access may allow for the delivery of strategies that can minimize disparities in vaccine uptake.

Literature has identified two categories of barriers, structural (physical) and informational, that may affect vaccine access in these populations [9]. Structural barriers may be defined as organizational issues that impede vaccine supply or accessibility such as limited vaccine access sites or inadequate access to transportation. Meanwhile, informational barriers can be characterized as barriers induced by information distribution and infrastructure that influence a patient's compliance with vaccination [9]. Vaccination rates in migrant communities have been studied, and some barriers to access identified by Crawshaw et al. (2022) in this community include: "language, literacy, and communication barriers, practical and legal barriers to accessing and delivering vaccination services, and service barriers such as lack of specific guidelines and knowledge of health-care professionals" [1].

Meeting accessibility needs requires fostering and implementing strategies that focus on vaccines that are readily available and affordable to all regardless of their socioeconomic status, race, level of education, or geographic location. Identifying and understanding these obstacles to vaccine access may allow for the formulation of plans that promote vaccine access and acceptance, leading to the ultimate goal of herd immunity.

8.1.3.1 Information Accessibility

Kuehn et al. identified several informational barriers impacting vaccine access, which included but are not limited to language barriers, vaccine hesitancy, politically-motivated skepticism, and primary news consumption via social media. Although informational barriers are difficult to overcome, acknowledgment of these barriers represents forward mobility toward effective change.

First, lack of awareness and provider recommendation of vaccination is one of the biggest barriers among these populations. Lack of promotion by healthcare providers may contribute to vaccine hesitancy and possibly decreased uptake [27]. Healthcare professionals should be updated on current vaccination guidelines and schedules and be encouraged to promote vaccination to patients. Furthermore, patient education programs led by healthcare professionals within a community as well as partnerships with community-based organizations may be implemented as a solution [28]. Additionally, language barriers may present as an obstacle for vaccination access. One study conducted by Quadri et al. showed that people with a language preference other than English had delayed vaccination uptake when compared to those with English proficiency [29]. Healthcare professionals should consider the provision of linguistically aligned vaccine information tailored to a patient's language preferences as this may allow for more effective communication, thus leading to an increase in vaccine information accessibility and uptake.

Moreover, primary news consumption received through social media may augment feelings of vaccine hesitancy and skepticism leading to decreased vaccine uptake. Anti-vaccine content is frequently shared on social media [30]. Prior research has shown that exposure to vaccine-critical websites and blogs negatively impacts vaccination willingness [31]. For example, through social media, individuals have the ability to spread medically inaccurate, biased information about health issues like HPV and HPV vaccination. This raises concerns, as it impedes the capacity for herd immunity against HPV to occur, leading to greater health inequities among certain populations, because misinformation may lead some to elect against vaccination. There is a need for healthcare providers to deliver medically accurate information. Health professionals should take advantage of relevant news events to foster positive conversations about vaccination on social media, and most importantly remember to keep the conversation going even when news coverage starts to subside. Additionally, vaccine safety concerns, potential side effects, and lack of efficacy were considered the most prevalent topics presented in anti-vaccine content. Health professionals can help promote vaccine uptake among populations against vaccination by focusing on these concerns and providing valuable vaccination education through social media [32].

Addressing Misinformation

Misinformation, defined as the unintentional dissemination of false information, and disinformation, defined as the deliberate spreading of false information, both contribute significantly to vaccine hesitancy and refusal [33]. One infamous example is the 1998 study conducted by Andrew Wakefield, which sought to falsely link the MMR vaccine to autism [34]. Despite the paper being retracted in 2010 and the author found to have purposely used fraudulent and misleading data, it has had a lasting impact on vaccination rates. One study showed that families that had a child with diagnosed autism were less likely to complete that child's vaccination series and less likely to vaccinate the child's younger siblings [35]. Safety concerns continue to be a major reason for parental vaccine hesitancy with parents believing that the vaccine can cause brain damage and autism, belief that serious side effects are common, as well as skepticism about the timing of the vaccinations and the amount of vaccinations administered simultaneously [4, 36]. This misinformation often spreads through social networks, including family members, co-workers, social media platforms, and even news outlets.

Similarly, the COVID-19 pandemic was riddled with misinformation that ultimately led to lower vaccination rates [37]. Social media and conspiracy theories played a significant role in disseminating false information, alongside mistrust in vaccines and misconceptions about the severity of COVID-19. This misinformation further fueled vaccine hesitancy and refusal, prolonging the pandemic's impact [38].

Despite the challenges posed by misinformation, healthcare providers can employ effective strategies to counteract myths and increase vaccine acceptance. Strategies such as emphasizing the scientific consensus on vaccine safety and efficacy, using humor, and providing warnings about misinformation were shown to be effective. Although healthcare providers commonly use educational material and debunk myths, those methods have yielded mixed results. It is essential to avoid communication strategies such as scare tactics and ignoring uncertainties about vaccines as it has been shown to increase vaccine refusal and can further entrench distrust among vaccine-hesitant individuals [39, 40].

8.1.3.2 Physical Accessibility

As previously stated, vaccination possesses the capacity to diminish mortality and morbidity by curtailing the spread of disease. However, physical barriers still remain as it relates to vaccine accessibility. These barriers may include underinsurance or lack of health insurance and lack of preventative care access, insufficient access to transportation, geographical barriers, and inadequate amounts of vaccination sites. In participants found living in rural communities, limited vaccination sites accounted for low vaccination rates. Compounding variables in this population consisted of lack of transportation and vaccine skepticism. Possible solutions at the community level may be to hold healthcare professional-led vaccination events in rural areas such as farms and factories or have healthcare providers go to the individual homes of residents and provide vaccines [9]. Solutions at the systematic level may implement incentives for physicians and other healthcare providers to work in rural areas consequently leading to the increase in preventative care and vaccination access. Furthermore, healthcare providers can implement vaccination practices that promote the use of single-dose vaccinations (such as single-dose COVID-19 immunization) to promote vaccine compliance and mitigate access barriers in populations with geographical and transportation barriers. Additionally, integrating the adult vaccine schedule with scheduled annual healthcare appointments can help reduce the transportation burden.

Potential cost barriers and lack of health insurance among these populations also present a challenging obstacle to vaccine access. A study conducted by Lu et al. showed that uninsured adults had significantly lower vaccination coverage when compared to insured individuals. Removing cost barriers to adult vaccination might improve vaccine access. In addition, the implementation of programs that provide free or reduced-cost vaccines to underinsured adults may also promote vaccine uptake. For example, Merck, the manufacturer of HPV, pneumococcal, and Hepatitis B vaccines, implemented a program that provides assistance to those who are uninsured and those with lower socioeconomic status (MPAP). Furthermore, a lack of insurance may lead to a lack of preventative care. It has been shown that individuals with regular physician visits are more likely to have received vaccine recommendations when compared to those who did not have regular physician visits. This may indicate that an increased number of physician visits may enable opportunities for vaccine education and access [41]. With this in mind, healthcare providers should make a conscious effort to facilitate patient contact and promote annual visits. Healthcare providers can also provide resources to uninsured patients and refer them to free clinics in the community that facilitate preventative care and vaccination programs.

8.2 Community-Based Immunization Efforts

8.2.1 Vaccination Campaigns and Supplementary Immunization Activities

One of the earliest documented vaccination campaigns was the Spanish Smallpox Vaccine Expedition, from 1803 to 1813 [42–44]. In addition to physician training to administer immunizations and the distribution of vaccines to more rural areas, the campaign featured festivities, music, theater, and the involvement of ecclesiastical leadership. For its time, the effort was immensely successful (at some points reaching 12,000 vaccinations per month), extending to various countries in South and Central America. The success of future vaccination campaigns is contingent upon a number of factors identified from historic immunization efforts, summarized by Mark and Rigau-Pérez [45] from World Health Organization findings:

> Current immunization programs must pursue high coverage of a clearly defined target population, manage a reliable logistics and transport system, employ trained health workers, reduce administrative and geographical barriers (with fixed and, if necessary, mobile delivery sites), and inform and motivate the population to make use of the vaccine. Some of the major lessons learned by the Expanded Programme on Immunization of the World Health Organization in the 1980s also include the following: personal involvement of political, religious, and social leadership mobilizes communities; communication is a critical component of a program and uses multiple channels (face-to-face, print, mass media) to deliver the message; staff training provides the technical skills for planning and management; successful programs have a process measure (coverage) as well as outcome indicator (disease incidence); disease surveillance helps focus efforts on areas of greatest risk; decentralization of resources, coupled with a national plan of action, permits more effective and rapid activities; research and development provide a technical basis for advancing program goals; unbalanced concerns over risks, and public apathy toward immunization, as disease incidence declines, must be countered everywhere.

In the following section, we discuss in greater detail some considerations and necessary context of some of these factors as applicable to community-based interventions for increasing vaccine education and uptake.

8.2.1.1 Identifying Community Leaders and Key Organizations

The public's distrust in the healthcare system has led to vaccine hesitancy. Considering the current climate, clinicians need to apply strategic measures for promoting vaccine campaigns and combating misinformation. One of the most effective strategies to advance vaccine uptake is to appeal to highly esteemed leaders and grassroots community-based advocates who have substantive footholds in the communities they serve [46, 47].

It is imperative that clinicians first survey the communities of interest to identify organizations such as the YMCA, faith groups, cultural centers, community clinics, local businesses, schools, and other impactful institutions within the community. From these groups, clinicians should identify leaders such as clergy persons, governmental officials, and grassroots advocates who represent the cultural and linguistic diversity of the communities [48]. For example, vaccine clinics held in partnership with ballroom icons and local drag events have been successful in immunizing members of local LGBTQ+ communities [49].

Once key points of community contact are identified, clinicians should extensively engage with community leaders to discuss vaccine campaign plans and goals. Establishing formidable relationships with community influencers provides an invaluable opportunity for health providers to understand how they can meet the needs of the community.

Additionally, clinicians can liaise with leaders to host community meetings aimed at discussing the risks and benefits of vaccines. This would provide an opportunity for health providers to listen to the concerns of community members and to gauge community dynamics. Forging connections at the basic grassroots level will eventually create avenues to leverage "bottom-up" strategies.

In promoting vaccine campaigns, clinicians should be mindful of blindly imposing their own desires on the community. The intention behind identifying key community leaders is to ensure that the approach of the vaccine campaign is community centered.

General Community Spaces

Community spaces generally refer to diverse environments where individuals or groups tend to congregate to interact, share resources, and partake in certain activities. These spaces foster a sense of trust in individuals due to them providing a safe environment, open communication, equity, and the general well-being of the community. These organizations have played vital roles in health promotions. They serve as a bridge between the community and government authorities including health officials. They are often partnered with health systems, which often enables them to have access to certain resources. These community spaces include but are not limited to community centers, schools, libraries, and nonprofit organizations such as YMCA [50].

The lack of trust in vaccines poses significant barriers to their acceptance and uptake. Community-based organizations (CBOs) have gained the trust of their community members. This will assist the CBOs in delivering health messaging such as vaccine information. Previous studies have demonstrated that due to the faith that the population places in these organizations, they have been able to address certain obstacles to vaccination [51, 52].

One of the greatest barriers to immunizations that community spaces can help overcome is the lack of accessibility. In an attempt to study the different ways to increase vaccine uptake among migrant communities, the researchers of a study discovered that convenient local clinics in the area encouraged underserved groups to get vaccinated. They discovered that having open access to vaccinations in walk-in clinics significantly improved their uptake. These walk-in clinics could be set up anywhere from community centers, local charities to food banks [1].

General community spaces play a dual role: they serve as venues where vaccinations can be administered while also serving as information hubs, offering insights into vaccine safety, efficacy, and more. In 2021, a survey conducted in England discovered that the hesitancy from obtaining a COVID-19 booster vaccine was due to limited knowledge and understanding about its safety and efficacy. The findings of the researchers suggest the need for community venues that could provide the proper vaccine information and address certain questions and concerns [17].

Schools are among the community-based institutions that have significantly enhanced vaccination rates. Research has proven a significant impact on vaccine uptake due to school-led vaccination-clinic programs. For instance, during the COVID-19 pandemic, a program was implemented by Seattle Public Schools (SPS) to increase vaccination rates, especially in children aged 5–11. Through the strategic messaging, school-located vaccination clinics, and school-led community engagement that were included in this program, there was an 80.3% increase in the overall vaccine series completion. School-led vaccination efforts have also played a role in increasing other vaccinations among students such as the influenza virus and the human papillomavirus [5].

The nonprofit organization YMCA prides itself as one of the leading nonprofit organizations that promptly respond to the specific needs of its communities. During the pandemic, they served as vaccination sites for some communities that lacked access to pharmacies, and they helped provide transportation to the vaccination settings. They went as far as providing free child care for families in an attempt to help with vaccinations.

During the peak of the COVID-19 pandemic, many major community-based organizations played significant roles in increasing vaccination rates including but not limited to the American Red Cross and Doctors Without Borders. These organizations, if not directly involved, at least indirectly helped with the vaccination efforts due to their collaborations and partnerships with health agencies.

Religious Spaces

Before discussing the role that religious leaders and faith-based places of gathering play in immunization campaigns and vaccine perceptions, it is important to first understand how religion may impact individual decision-making with respect to being immunized. It is well-documented that, due to religious reasons, some individuals may refrain from vaccination for themselves, dependent minors, and/or those for whom they act as healthcare proxy [53]. Individuals' experience of religious choices can be understood as a product of sociocultural background as well as religious canon. It is worth acknowledging the complex interplay between religion and culture with regard to vaccination intention; there have been instances where individuals may believe their religion prohibits immunization—due to an understanding of faith-based practice imparted by a cultural upbringing—but religious canon may in fact permit, if not encourage, immunizations. A notable example can be seen in documented vaccine hesitancy in the Muslim community, which has been the subject of multiple international studies [54]. Concern about whether certain vaccines contain animal products or are animal-derived seems to be a large contributing factor to vaccine perceptions in this group; however, Islamic scholarly consensus is that immunization, as a form of attending to personal health and supporting community well-being, is strongly recommended if not a religious obligation. Similar concerns about ingredients exist in other religious demographics: members of the Jewish community have expressed worries in the past about which vaccines are kosher/free of components of porcine origin, and some individuals of specific Hindu sects require that vaccines are free of components of bovine origin [55, 56].

Another reason an individual may object to vaccination may occur when the process by which ingredients were sourced/produced is not aligned with their religious values. Some individuals oppose some immunizations on the basis that historic fetal cell lines were used in the production and manufacturing process, concerns leveled most prominently at the COVID-19 vaccine [57–59]. Notably, a number of faith-based anti-abortion groups were vocal in their support of COVID-19 vaccines, emphasizing alongside medical experts that vaccines themselves contained no fetal cells/fetal cell components.

Individuals belonging to a given faith may express a willingness to receive vaccinations but uptake may be precluded by specific religious concerns. Even in cases where there is ambiguity in a religion about vaccines, bringing to an individual's attention that ambiguity exists may allow them to make a more informed decision with more personal agency. Religious leaders, clergy, and scholars play a pivotal role in influencing vaccine perceptions and uptake in their communities by virtue of their clerical training, experience with community work, and the goodwill held in them by constituents and peers. Additionally, sharing medical expertise with religious leaders allows them to form more informed opinions/rulings and take part in advocacy more effectively. It is imperative that vaccine initiatives identify and include individuals who hold leadership roles in religious communities and enlist their aid in dispelling misconceptions about vaccination that may be held by community members and in organizing effective immunization programs [60]. It is worth noting that physical religious spaces/places of worship are not only well-trusted but also frequented and accessible to individuals who attend their services, often behaving as important third spaces for historically marginalized communities [61, 62]. It follows that interventions in religious spaces can have a significant impact on vaccine uptake and community awareness of the utility of immunizations.

8.2.1.2 Specific Community-Based Organization Initiatives and Outcomes

The need for diverse tools and strategies to increase vaccine rates has yet to be dissipated. There have been multiple initiatives designed by community-based organizations to increase vaccination rates that have proven to be successful [63, 64].

Community-driven interventions are essential for making a significant impact on vaccination rates as emphasized by four UNICEF-supported interventions. These interventions were adopted by four different countries to boost the acceptance and demand for COVID-19 vaccines during the pandemic. Most of these countries had a slow uptake of the vaccines prior to their interventions. Zambia utilized *Community Rapid Assessments* to attain knowledge of the people's perceptions and behaviors regarding the vaccine. The approach they employed included rapid assessments in the form of mobile surveys that were available to adults who opted into them. They were able to identify population segments that had shared beliefs and motivations regarding the COVID-19 vaccine. They were then able to utilize these newly acquired insights to develop strategies that addressed the specific needs of individuals with different persona types in the population.

As for Iraq, the Ministry of Health of Iraq partnered with UNICEF to develop their approach titled *3IS (Intensification of Integrated Immunization) outreach.* This approach was implemented for both the COVID-19 vaccine and the routine immunizations. This initiative was designed to be flexible. The outreach teams utilized a mobile clinic and engaged individuals in diverse general community spaces such as shopping centers, public parks, and schools. In the span of 10 months, they administered over 4.4 million doses of combined COVID-19 and routine immunization vaccines. Among them, there were 149,000 children who had not yet commenced any of the routine immunizations. This initiative had a dual success in both delivering health messages and immunizing.

Ghana's initiative to improve COVID-19 vaccination uptake included applying a *Human-Centered design (HCD).* Their approach aimed to identify the human factors that surrounded the low vaccine uptake in Ghana. The findings suggested that many individuals in that population were not against getting vaccinated as long as the opportunity and process to do so was an easy one. Through the human-centered design approach, communication and messages regarding vaccines were improved. Strategies were developed to make the vaccination services easily accessible and convenient for those who were willing to accept them.

India also launched their community-led COLLECT R-CCE initiative, which stands for *Risk Communication and Community Engagement.* The specific actions in this program were community-led awareness campaigns in which they educated individuals regarding the vaccines, dispelled myths and rumors, and promoted vaccination. They also utilized door-to-door interactions to build awareness. Through this program, they accomplished improvements in public health response and reduced vaccine hesitancy. Additionally, vaccination rates increased by 25% [52].

Other initiatives that have been implemented by diverse community-based organizations include the use of multilingual staff members to reach diverse populations, manual outreach programs, and centralized reminder/recall systems.

8.2.2 Community and Outpatient Pharmacy

In all 50 states and Washington D. C., pharmacists are authorized to administer vaccines; however, laws vary from state to state regarding which vaccines pharmacists can administer, patient age restrictions, and whether or not a protocol with a local prescriber or a prescription is needed to immunize [65]. Throughout the years, pharmacists have been considered one of the most trusted and accessible healthcare professionals. With this distinction, pharmacists have emerged over the past few decades as an integral part of the immunization movement, even being recognized by the CDC. In a recent meta-analysis, pharmacist involvement as immunizers and/or advocators significantly increased immunization rates, especially with the influenza vaccine in the United States as well as other high-income countries [66]. As commercial health insurance, Medicare, and Medicaid have continued to broaden their vaccine coverage, pharmacists, pharmacy interns, and pharmacy technicians have maintained optimal training to ensure high-quality immunization recommendations and injection techniques. Currently, pharmacists, pharmacy interns, and pharmacy technicians require training and certification prior to administering immunizations. Oftentimes, this occurs through the American Pharmacists Association Pharmacy-Based Immunization Delivery Program, which is a combination of self-study, live lecture, and an assessment of immunization technique [67]. Additionally, immunization continuing education tends to be a requirement of many pharmacist and pharmacy technician license renewals. With the evolution of pharmacist-administered vaccines progressing since the early 1990s, pharmacists were poised and ready to begin immunizing against COVID-19. As of August 2023, over 300 million doses of the COVID-19 vaccine have been administered by the Federal Pharmacy Program [68].

The American Pharmacists Association places a strong emphasis on immunization advocacy, with core themes centering around prevention, partnerships, quality, documentation, and empowerment. Disease state prevention is key as pharmacists can serve as educators, facilitators, and immunizers, especially in providing education, debunking vaccine myths, and reducing vaccine hesitancy. Being one of the most accessible healthcare professionals allows pharmacists to provide this education to patients, caregivers, and even other healthcare providers; this accessibility has been identified as an important avenue of reaching underserved patient populations, particularly through community pharmacy settings [69]. Prior to legislation passing for pharmacists to administer immunizations, housing immunizers within community pharmacies was a great way to promote immunizations and provide access. Additionally, in many states, pharmacists are unable to administer vaccines to children under 3 years of age, so the facilitation and promotion of immunizations are key in this patient population. Partnerships are so incredibly important as physician offices and community pharmacies often do not carry all available vaccines, especially travel vaccines, so partnerships with local health departments are vital to ensuring patients know where to obtain these necessary vaccines. Additionally, partnerships with skilled nursing facilities, universities, faith-based organizations, and businesses allow pharmacists to administer vaccines on-site as part of health and wellness initiatives. When referring to quality and documentation, these go hand and hand to ensure pharmacists, pharmacy interns, and pharmacy technicians maintain a high level of training and continuing education and also ensure accurate documentation within the community pharmacy, statewide immunizations database, and in the Vaccine Adverse Event Reporting System (VAERS) if necessary [67].

8.2.3 Mobilization and Training for Nonphysician Vaccinators

While all immunizing healthcare professionals have varying authority as it pertains to immunizations, the key factor is to abide by the laws and regulations within their respective state of practice. Some healthcare professions may not need immunization certifications as it is considered within their scope of practice while others require some external training, like pharmacists [70, 71]. Regardless, it is vital to be up-to-date with the recommendations of the CDC's Advisory Committee on

Immunization Practices (ACIP) that are published annually as well as any updates in the interim. Additionally, some healthcare professions require continuing education regarding vaccinations within a respective renewal time period.

As seen during the COVID-19 pandemic, vaccine recommendations change and laws will often change along with it. In many states, pharmacists were not permitted to immunize children; however, as COVID-19 vaccine Emergency Use Authorizations expanded to include children, regulations barring pharmacist-administered immunizations in this patient population changed as well. Additionally, many states authorized pharmacy technicians to administer certain vaccines under a pharmacist's supervision as a result of the increased immunization need and approved training programs targeting pharmacy technicians. In Spring 2021, the U.S. Department of Health & Human Services authorized medical students and other health professions students with training and adequate supervision to administer COVID-19 vaccines as part of efforts to preclude the spread of the virus and variants within the country [72].

All healthcare professionals have a role to play in the promotion of immunizations but the first step is truly feeling comfortable administering vaccines. While immunizers may have different roles whether it be solely administering the vaccine or additionally recommending/choosing the correct vaccine for a patient, the only way to feel more comfortable with this task is to continue keeping up this skill and practicing at the top of one's license.

8.3 Looking Forward

It is evident that barriers to immunization have their roots in complex structural factors, with doubt and misinformation about vaccines being spread through social interactions across various settings. It stands to reason that adequate solutions to such public health issues lie in cultivating community partnerships and enacting multifactorial interventions in the very social settings where vaccine hesitancy may begin. These efforts are not possible without the active participation of healthcare professionals—clinicians armed not only with expertise with vaccinations themselves but also with increased cultural awareness and empathy for the many reasons why an individual may feel trepidation about being immunized. We hope that this chapter has been helpful to clinicians and trainees in achieving that goal.

References

1. Crawshaw AF, Farah Y, Deal A, et al. Defining the determinants of vaccine uptake and undervaccination in migrant populations in Europe to improve routine and COVID-19 vaccine uptake: a systematic review. Lancet Infect Dis. 2022;22:e254. https://doi.org/10.1016/s1473-3099(22)00066-4.

2. World Health Organization. Catch-up vaccination. World Health Organization; 2021b. https://www.who.int/teams/immunization-vaccines-and-biologicals/essential-programme-on-immunization/implementation/catch-up-vaccination. Accessed 8 Aug 2024.
3. Ekezie W, Awwad S, Krauchenberg A, et al. Access to vaccination among disadvantaged, isolated and difficult-to-reach communities in the WHO european region: a systematic review. Vaccines. 2022;10:1038. https://doi.org/10.3390/vaccines10071038.
4. McGregor S, Goldman RD. Determinants of parental vaccine hesitancy. Canad Fam Phys. 2021;67:339–41. https://doi.org/10.46747/cfp.6705339.
5. Fairlie T, Chu B, Thomas ES, et al. School-based interventions to increase student COVID-19 vaccination coverage in public school populations with low coverage – Seattle, Washington, December 2021–June 2022. MMWR Morb Mortal Wkly Rep. 2023;72:283–7. https://doi.org/10.15585/mmwr.mm7211a3.
6. Khalili D, Caplan A. Off the grid: vaccinations among homeschooled children. J Law Med Ethics. 2007;35:471–7. https://doi.org/10.1111/j.1748-720x.2007.00169.x.
7. O'Leary ST, Opel DJ, Cataldi JR, et al. Strategies for improving vaccine communication and uptake. Pediatrics. 2024; https://doi.org/10.1542/peds.2023-065483.
8. Centers for Disease Control and Prevention. Vaccine administration protocols. Centers for Disease Control and Prevention; 2018. https://www.cdc.gov/vaccines/hcp/admin/admin-protocols.html. Accessed 9 Aug 2024.
9. Kuehn M, LaMori J, DeMartino JK, et al. Assessing barriers to access and equity for COVID-19 vaccination in the US. BMC Publ Health. 2022;22(1):2263. Published 2022 Dec 3. https://doi.org/10.1186/s12889-022-14636-1.
10. Nuwarda RF, Ramzan I, Weekes L, Kayser V. Vaccine hesitancy: contemporary issues and historical background. Vaccines (Basel). 2022;10(10):1595. Published 2022 Sep 22. https://doi.org/10.3390/vaccines10101595.
11. Patel P. Forced sterilization of women as discrimination. Publ Health Rev. 2017;38(1) https://doi.org/10.1186/s40985-017-0060-9.
12. Heintzelman CA. The Tuskegee syphilis study and its implications for the 21st century. The New Social Worker. 2003;10(4):4–5.
13. DeStefano F, Bodenstab HM, Offit PA. Principal controversies in vaccine safety in the United States. Clin Infect Dis. 2019;69(4):726–31. https://doi.org/10.1093/cid/ciz135.
14. Qian M, Chou S-Y, Lai EK. Confirmatory bias in health decisions: evidence from the MMR-autism controversy. J Health Econ. 2020;70:102284. https://doi.org/10.1016/j.jhealeco.2019.102284.
15. Millman AJ, Denson DJ, Allen ML, et al. A health equity approach for implementation of JYNNEOS vaccination at large, community-based LGBTQIA+ events – Georgia, August 27–September 5, 2022. MMWR Morb Mortal Wkly Rep. 2022;71:1382–883. https://doi.org/10.15585/mmwr.mm7143e4.
16. Stacey K. The fight to overcome vaccine hesitancy among African Americans. Financial Times; 2021. https://www.ft.com/content/515d3949-4379-42db-aa69-f11ffa116e39. Accessed 10 Aug 2024.
17. Meyer C, Goffe L, Antonopoulou V, et al. Using the precaution adoption process model to understand decision-making about the COVID-19 booster vaccine in England. Vaccine. 2023;41:2466–75. https://doi.org/10.1016/j.vaccine.2023.02.047.
18. Navin MC, Wasserman JA, Ahmad M, Bies S. Vaccine education, reasons for refusal, and vaccination behavior. Am J Prev Med. 2019;56:359–67. https://doi.org/10.1016/j.amepre.2018.10.024.
19. Brunson EK, Buttenheim A, Omer S, Quinn SC. Strategies for building confidence in the covid-19 vaccines. National Academies Press; 2021. https://doi.org/10.17226/26068.
20. Powell M. Promoting vaccination: the right approach for the right group. NIHR Evidence; 2024. https://evidence.nihr.ac.uk/collection/promoting-vaccination-the-right-approach-for-the-right-group/. Accessed 8 Aug 2024.

21. Edwards JG, Cheston CC, Kelly CA, et al. A community-based COVID-19 vaccine education initiative. Pediatrics. 2022; https://doi.org/10.1542/peds.2022-057374.
22. Robinson R, Nguyen E, Wright M, et al. Factors contributing to vaccine hesitancy and reduced vaccine confidence in rural underserved populations. Human Soc Sci Commun. 2022;9(1) https://doi.org/10.1057/s41599-022-01439-3.
23. Nowak GJ, Shen AK, Schwartz JL. Using campaigns to improve perceptions of the value of adult vaccination in the United States: health communication considerations and insights. Vaccine. 2017;35:5543–50. https://doi.org/10.1016/j.vaccine.2017.08.064.
24. Lu PJ, Hung MC, Srivastav A, et al. Surveillance of vaccination coverage among adult populations -United States, 2018. MMWR Surveill Summ. 2021;70(3):1–26. Published 2021 May 14. https://doi.org/10.15585/mmwr.ss7003a1.
25. Evans D, Norrbom C, Schmidt S, et al. Engaging community-based organizations to address barriers in public health programs: lessons learned from covid-19 vaccine acceptance programs in diverse rural communities. Health Secur. 2023;21:S17. https://doi.org/10.1089/hs.2023.0017.
26. Bedford H, Attwell K, Danchin M, Marshall H, Corben P, Leask J. Vaccine hesitancy, refusal and access barriers: the need for clarity in terminology. Vaccine. 2018;36(44):6556–8. https://doi.org/10.1016/j.vaccine.2017.08.004.
27. Cartmell KB, Young-Pierce J, McGue S, et al. Barriers, facilitators, and potential strategies for increasing HPV vaccination: a statewide assessment to inform action. Papillomavirus Res. 2018;5:21–31. https://doi.org/10.1016/j.pvr.2017.11.003.
28. U.S. Department of Health & Human Services. 3 ways community-based organizations can promote COVID-19 vaccination. COVID.gov; 2023. https://www.covid.gov/resource/3-ways-community-based-organizations-can-promote-covid-19-vaccination. Accessed 9 Aug 2024.
29. Quadri NS, Knowlton G, Vazquez Benitez G, et al. Evaluation of preferred language and timing of COVID-19 vaccine uptake and disease outcomes. JAMA Netw Open. 2023; https://doi.org/10.1001/jamanetworkopen.2023.7877.
30. Oehler RL. On measles, vaccination, social media activism and how to win back our role as our patients' best advocates. Clin Infect Dis. 2019; https://doi.org/10.1093/cid/ciz656.
31. Betsch C, Renkewitz F, Betsch T, Ulshöfer C. The influence of vaccine-critical websites on perceiving vaccination risks. J Health Psychol. 2010;15(3):446–55. https://doi.org/10.1177/1359105309353647.
32. Ortiz RR, Smith A, Coyne-Beasley T. A systematic literature review to examine the potential for social media to impact HPV vaccine uptake and awareness, knowledge, and attitudes about HPV and HPV vaccination. Hum Vaccin Immunother. 2019;15(7–8):1465–75. https://doi.org/10.1080/21645515.2019.1581543.
33. CSI Library. Misinformation and disinformation: thinking critically about information sources. CUNY College of Staten Island Library; 2021.
34. Sathyanarayana Rao T, Andrade C. The MMR vaccine and autism: sensation, refutation, retraction, and fraud. Indian J Psychiatr. 2011;53:95. https://doi.org/10.4103/0019-5545.82529.
35. Zerbo O, Modaressi S, Goddard K, et al. Vaccination patterns in children after autism spectrum disorder diagnosis and in their younger siblings. JAMA Pediatr. 2018;172:469. https://doi.org/10.1001/jamapediatrics.2018.0082.
36. McKee C, Bohannon K. Exploring the reasons behind parental refusal of vaccines. J Pediatr Pharmacol Therap. 2016;21:104–9. https://doi.org/10.5863/1551-6776-21.2.104.
37. Loomba S, de Figueiredo A, Piatek SJ, et al. Measuring the impact of COVID-19 vaccine misinformation on vaccination intent in the UK and USA. Nat Human Behav. 2021;5:337–48. https://doi.org/10.1038/s41562-021-01056-1.
38. Zhao S, Hu S, Zhou X, et al. The prevalence, features, influencing factors, and solutions for COVID-19 vaccine misinformation: systematic review. JMIR Publ Health Surveil. 2023; https://doi.org/10.2196/40201.

39. Finney Rutten LJ, Zhu X, Leppin AL, et al. Evidence-based strategies for clinical organizations to address COVID-19 vaccine hesitancy. Mayo Clin Proc. 2021;96:699–707. https://doi.org/10.1016/j.mayocp.2020.12.024.
40. Whitehead HS, French CE, Caldwell DM, et al. A systematic review of communication interventions for countering vaccine misinformation. Vaccine. 2023;41:1018–34. https://doi.org/10.1016/j.vaccine.2022.12.059.
41. Lu P, O'Halloran A, Williams WW. Impact of health insurance status on vaccination coverage among adult populations. Am J Prevent Med. 2015;48(6):647–61. https://doi.org/10.1016/j.amepre.2014.12.008.
42. World Health Organization. History of smallpox vaccination. Google Arts & Culture; 2020. https://artsandculture.google.com/story/qAURxyAnf5tcXg. Accessed 10 Aug 2024.
43. World Health Organization. A brief history of vaccination. World Health Organization; 2021a. https://www.who.int/news-room/spotlight/history-of-vaccination/a-brief-history-of-vaccination. Accessed 10 Aug 2024.
44. World Health Organization. Immunization campaigns. World Health Organization; 2023. https://www.who.int/teams/immunization-vaccines-and-biologicals/essential-programme-on-immunization/implementation/immunization-campaigns. Accessed 8 Aug 2024.
45. Mark C, Rigau-Pérez JG. The world's first immunization campaign: the Spanish smallpox vaccine expedition, 1803–1813. Bull Hist Med. 2009;83:63–94. https://doi.org/10.1353/bhm.0.0173.
46. Community Preventive Services Task Force. Vaccination programs: community-based interventions implemented in combination. The Community Guide; 2023. https://www.thecommunityguide.org/findings/vaccination-programs-community-based-interventions-implemented-combination.html. Accessed 9 Aug 2024.
47. Shen AK, Browne S, Srivastava T, et al. Trusted messengers and trusted messages: the role for community-based organizations in promoting COVID-19 and routine immunizations. Vaccine. 2023;41:1994–2002. https://doi.org/10.1016/j.vaccine.2023.02.045.
48. Centers for Disease Control and Prevention. Partnering for vaccine equity. Centers for Disease Control and Prevention; 2024. https://www.cdc.gov/vaccines/health-equity/index.html. Accessed 8 Aug 2024.
49. Singer RB, Crooks N, Singer R, et al. Ballroom icons and the power to promote covid-19 vaccination among black and Brown LGBTQ+ individuals. Am J Public Health. 2022;112:17–20. https://doi.org/10.2105/ajph.2021.306581.
50. Dhaliwal BK, Seth R, Thankachen B, et al. Leading from the frontlines: community-oriented approaches for strengthening vaccine delivery and acceptance. BMC Proc. 2023;17:5. https://doi.org/10.1186/s12919-023-00259-w.
51. DiVirgilio L, Boshara A, Hunt BR, et al. A community-informed approach to COVID-19 vaccine roll-out in under-served areas in Chicago. Front Public Health. 2022; https://doi.org/10.3389/fpubh.2022.863125.
52. Hopkins KL, Underwood T, Iddrisu I, et al. Community-based approaches to increase COVID-19 vaccine uptake and demand: lessons learned from four UNICEF-supported interventions. Vaccine. 2023;11:1180. https://doi.org/10.3390/vaccines11071180.
53. Maine Chapter American Academy of Pediatrics, Religious Views of Vaccination At-A-Glance; 2011.
54. Alsuwaidi AR, Hammad HA, Elbarazi I, Sheek-Hussein M. Vaccine hesitancy within the Muslim Community: Islamic faith and Public Health Perspectives. Hum Vaccin Immunother. 2023;19 https://doi.org/10.1080/21645515.2023.2190716.
55. Institute for Vaccine Safety. Religion and vaccines – institute for vaccine safety. Johns Hopkins Bloomberg School of Public Health Institute for Vaccine Safety; 2022. https://www.vaccinesafety.edu/religion-and-vaccines/. Accessed 10 Aug 2024
56. State of Oregon Health Authority. Vaccine facts for Hindu faith communities. State of Oregon Health Authority; 2021.

57. Amin AB, Bednarczyk RA, Ray CE, et al. Association of moral values with vaccine hesitancy. Nat Hum Behav. 2017;1:873–80. https://doi.org/10.1038/s41562-017-0256-5.
58. Grabenstein JD. What the world's religions teach, applied to vaccines and immune globulins. Vaccine. 2013;31:2011–23. https://doi.org/10.1016/j.vaccine.2013.02.026.
59. Suzia A, Barella A, Barella S, et al. A Christian statement on vaccination and religious objection; 2019.
60. Rabin BA, Cain KL, Watson P, et al. Scaling and sustaining COVID-19 vaccination through meaningful community engagement and care coordination for underserved communities: hybrid type 3 effectiveness-implementation sequential multiple assignment randomized trial. Implement Sci. 2023;18:28. https://doi.org/10.1186/s13012-023-01283-2.
61. How vaccines protect communities. Penn Medicine. https://www.pennmedicine.org/news/news-blog/2021/march/how-vaccines-protect-communities. Accessed 10 Aug 2024.
62. Finlay J, Esposito M, Kim MH, et al. Closure of 'third places'? exploring potential consequences for collective health and Wellbeing. Health Place. 2019;60:102225. https://doi.org/10.1016/j.healthplace.2019.102225.
63. LeBaron CW, Starnes D, Dini EF, et al. The impact of interventions by a community-based organization on inner-city vaccination coverage. Arch Pediatr Adolesc Med. 1998;152:327. https://doi.org/10.1001/archpedi.152.4.327.
64. Office of Disease Prevention and Health Promotion. Vaccination programs: community-based interventions implemented in combination. U.S. Department of Health & Human Services; 2014. https://health.gov/healthypeople/tools-action/browse-evidence-based-resources/vaccination-programs-community-based-interventions-implemented-combination. Accessed 8 Aug 2024.
65. National Alliance of State Pharmacy Associations. Pharmacist immunization authority. NASPA; 2023. https://naspa.us/blog/resource/pharmacist-authority-to-immunize/. Accessed 9 Aug 2024.
66. Le LM, Veettil SK, Donaldson D, et al. The impact of pharmacist involvement on immunization uptake and other outcomes: an updated systematic review and meta-analysis. J Am Pharm Assoc. 2022;62:1499. https://doi.org/10.1016/j.japh.2022.06.008.
67. American Pharmacists Association, National Alliance of State Pharmacy Associations. Pharmacist Administered Vaccines; 2023.
68. Centers for Disease Control & Prevention. Covid-19 vaccination federal retail pharmacy partnership program. Centers for Disease Control and Prevention; 2023. https://archive.cdc.gov/www_cdc_gov/vaccines/covid-19/retail-pharmacy-program/index.html. Accessed 10 Aug 2024.
69. Kirkdale CL, Nebout G, Megerlin F, Thornley T. Benefits of pharmacist-led flu vaccination services in community pharmacy. Ann Pharm Fr. 2017;75:3–8. https://doi.org/10.1016/j.pharma.2016.08.005.
70. Bach A, Goad J. The role of community pharmacy-based vaccination in the USA: current practice and future directions. Integr Pharm Res Pract. 2015;67 https://doi.org/10.2147/iprp.s63822.
71. Hogue MD, Grabenstein JD, Foster SL, Rothholz MC. Pharmacist involvement with immunizations: a decade of professional advancement. J Am Pharm Assoc. 2006;46:168–82. https://doi.org/10.1331/154434506776180621.
72. The White House. Fact sheet: president Biden expands efforts to recruit more vaccinators. The White House; 2021. https://www.whitehouse.gov/briefing-room/statements-releases/2021/03/12/fact-sheet-president-biden-expands-efforts-to-recruit-more-vaccinators/. Accessed 9 Aug 2024.

Chapter 9
Vaccine Hesitancy in Diverse Communities: A Holistic Approach to Patient-Centered Care

Farzanna S. Haffizulla

9.1 Introduction

The impact of effective, empathic interpersonal communication in healthcare is paramount to improving patient outcomes. Clinicians' communication and connection with their patients start well before patients enter the clinical space, such as in an office setting, hospital, telemedicine visit, etc. The clinical experience is integrally connected to all patients' clinical care journeys. This includes, but is not limited to, digital communication through electronic medical record reminders, social media reviews, and nonclinical interactions with staff and personnel through various media such as phones, practice apps, and emails. In addition, easy digital access to elements of our work and lives plays a role in a patient's assessment of clinicians. This complex interplay of factors contributes to a patient's embrace, adherence, or action in relation to a clinician's recommendations. These factors include cultural nuances, biases, an individual's perspectives, social determinants of health, and trust. This chapter outlines cultural humility and social determinants of health (SDOH) as critical factors in healthcare communication in addressing vaccine hesitation. This will include an overview of psychological and relevant person-specific social determinants of health, socioeconomic factors contributing to hesitancy, and potential communication strategies, best practices, and future directions.

F. S. Haffizulla (✉)
Nova Southeastern University Dr. Kiran C. Patel College of Osteopathic Medicine, Fort Lauderdale, FL, USA
e-mail: fhaffizull@nova.edu

A. J. Chase et al. (eds.), *Vaccine Hesitancy Curriculum*,
https://doi.org/10.1007/978-3-031-88668-3_9

9.2 Understanding Vaccine Hesitancy

According to the World Health Organization's Strategic Advisory Group of Experts on Immunization (SAGE) [1].

> … hesitancy is a behavioral phenomenon which is vaccine and context-specific and measured against an expectation of reaching a specific vaccination coverage goal, given the immunization services available. Vaccine hesitancy may be present in situations where vaccination uptake is low because of system failures, e.g. stock-outs, limited availability of vaccination services (time, place, etc.), curtailment of vaccine services in the presence of conflict or natural disaster, but in these situations, hesitancy is not the main explanation for the presence of unvaccinated or under-vaccinated members of the population. Assessing whether hesitancy is present in a population and differentiating hesitancy from other reasons why children/adults are unvaccinated or under-vaccinated is essential for the selection of interventions needed to address low vaccine uptake.

In contrast to hesitancy, vaccine apathy can be a precursor to hesitancy but with no psychological investment [1].

In this chapter, I will describe vaccine hesitancy in communities of color, primarily focusing on Black, Caribbean, and Hispanic populations. I take a two-pronged approach—pairing existing research-derived data with extrapolated recommendations. The World Health Organization's Behavioral and Social Drivers of Vaccination Framework creates a guide for discussion in this chapter. This guide allows for deeper questioning and discussion around many "unknowns" that significantly impact a decision to get vaccinated, such as internal thoughts, feelings, motivation, and external variables, inclusive of social and practical issues [2, 3].

9.3 The Intersection of the Past and Present

Historically, communities of color developed a mistrust of the healthcare system and research from notorious studies like the Study of Syphilis in Tuskegee, Alabama [4], Dr. Marion Sims' experiments of enslaved women [5], and the well-known story about the unethical use of Henrietta Lacks' breast cancer cells. In these experiments, Black people and many other peoples of color (POC) endured significant torture, pain, abuse, mistreatment, and harm. The lasting effects of these horrific ordeals, coupled with structural racism and biases baked into our medical system, create a vicious cycle of mistrust, health disparities, and poor patient outcomes. In the public health arena, people of color have endured countless injustices, inhumane treatment, and oppression [6]. It is vital to recognize that the inequities and injustices that exist today perpetuate, amplify, and contribute to ongoing mistrust in the healthcare system in the United States.

The COVID-19 pandemic magnified existing disparities in marginalized populations. Newman et al., in their scoping review of COVID-19 vaccine hesitancy and undervaccination among marginalized populations in the United States and Canada, identified structural racism/stigma and institutional mistrust as leading causes, followed by vaccine safety, side effects, trust in individual healthcare providers, and perceived infection risk as influencing factors. Structural factors such as poor vaccine access/availability, structural racism/stigma, lack of paid sick days, insufficient digital technology access, and long distance from vaccine access points without transportation were also critical contributors. Inadequate culturally and linguistically appropriate resources were also notable factors [7]. The COVID-19 pandemic not only further magnified disparities but also vaccination hesitancy. In fact, according to the results published by Willis et al. in Preventive Medicine, "We found experiences of racial discrimination are associated with greater odds of COVID-19 vaccine hesitancy even after adjusting for sociodemographic characteristics, political affiliation, prior COVID-19 infection, and having a primary care doctor. For every one-unit increase in racial discrimination across one's lifetime, we found a 4% increase in the odds of COVID-19 vaccine hesitancy. The total increase in odds could be substantially higher depending on the lifetime frequency of experiences of racial discrimination. These findings are consistent with the limited body of research examining racial discrimination and COVID-19 vaccine hesitancy, as well as the limited work linking racial disparities in vaccination rates with structural racism" [8–10].

During the pandemic, I served as principal investigator of a federally funded research study, *Advancing Health Literacy in the City of Lauderhill to Enhance Equitable Community Responses to COVID-19*, with the goal of improving COVID-19 health literacy and vaccination among Black, Jamaican, Haitian, and Hispanic residents in the City of Lauderhill, Florida. Lauderhill includes 8.5 square miles of Broward County, Florida, and is designated by the US Housing and Urban Development (HUD) as low-income. According to the City's 2021 Community Needs Assessment, the population is almost 75,000, of which 85% are racial/ethnic minorities. The overall social vulnerability index is high at 0.76 [22]. One of our aims was to determine the reasons for vaccine hesitancy [11]. Our curated data collection tools included surveys and focus groups designed to amplify the voices of the community we served. We engaged over 2000 city residents, business owners, and leaders in this study. Community residents were actively engaged in co-creating culturally tailored health education materials and in outreach to their networks of clients, friends, and family members for inclusion in our study. My work on community initiatives with the City of Lauderhill predated the start of this study by a few years, allowing for trust and relationship building to serve as a nidus for our work together. We found that a significant portion of the respondents who did not take the vaccine expressed concerns about the safety of the COVID-19 vaccines, indicating a potential barrier to their acceptance and uptake. Additionally, many respondents did not perceive COVID-19 as a significant threat to their health, suggesting a perception of low personal risk. These factors mirror the findings noted in the studies above [11].

Moreover, doubts about the vaccine's effectiveness in providing protection against COVID-19 were expressed by a considerable portion of the respondents. The influence of family members who discouraged vaccination, unfamiliarity with vaccination locations, and limited access due to restricted opening hours of vaccination sites were also reported as obstacles to receiving the vaccine. Furthermore, some individuals cited underlying medical conditions, religious or cultural reasons, or simply not having a specific reason contributing to their decision against vaccination. These findings highlight the diverse range of reasons behind vaccine hesitancy or refusal, emphasizing the importance of collaborative communication and interventions or initiatives to address these concerns and promote vaccination coverage. Interestingly, residents found the COVID-19 information flyers informative and engaging, but their willingness to take action based on the information provided was lower than expected.

Initial thoughts about vaccine usage were mostly negative, citing hesitancy and concerns about vaccine development being "rushed," perceived feelings of being forced to get vaccinated, and previous experience with other shots. Those who did not receive the vaccine at the time of the focus group interviews indicated a variety of different reasons for not getting vaccinated, including not wanting to give into "peer pressure," skepticism about vaccine effectiveness, lack of knowledge about long-term side effects, and perceptions that either there was not enough information available or there was conflicting information that created a cause to pause. A non-Hispanic black female from Jamaica questioned vaccine effectiveness after her father, who was vaccinated and boosted, was infected with COVID-19:

> *I didn't take the vaccine still because I, I just you know, thought I could fight it. But my dad kept urging us to, you know, get it. And he actually took the booster and the other. [...] He took all of them but still got COVID. And I was like, "Wait, isn't the vaccine like, supposed to prevent him from getting it?" Then he still got it?*

Some participants expressed mistrust. A Hispanic Black Caribbean female stated:

> *I felt like things were progressing so quickly. And there was so much information being put out there. And I felt like in general, I feel that the people were getting so much information, that there was an automatic mistrust with not just the medical system, but also the government.*

Some participants liked having information available on different media types, such as email, podcasts, text messaging, local news, radio, and social media. Subthemes that emerged were that not everyone is a consumer of the same media (e.g., listens to the radio, watches the news on television, is active on social media, etc.), so it is important to utilize multiple media outlets/types. Another subtheme that emerged was tailoring messages and methods to specific age groups, outlining different approaches for different age groups (e.g., textual information for seniors, youth teaching parents/adults, and young people on social media platforms). A non-Hispanic Black Haitian female mentioned that children should be taught about COVID-19 in schools so they can come home and educate their parents:

> *If the kid is very educated, and they're doing it respectfully. I do think some parents will sit back and listen because I do think it comes to a point where sometimes your kids know more than you. And you're like, wait, no, they're making sense.*

There were also various responses regarding suggestions for who should be sharing COVID-19 information. However, there was a subtheme of having reputable, educated, and "genuine" individuals with factual information. This included health professionals, local community leaders, entertainers/personalities, different people in social networks, and family members. A trusted source or person is certainly not a universal choice by members of the same community. In fact, a Hispanic-Black female shared some skepticism about religious leaders sharing information:

> *I may trust my local pastor, but then where is he getting his information from? And I won't trust any of these TV pastors, because where are you getting your information from? You're definitely getting paid to do this at this point. So, I would in this sense, I would go more with the government leaders in the doctors because even with being religious, I do believe that the Lord has appointed certain people for certain positions, everyone doesn't belong everywhere.*

One word that was repeated across focus groups was "genuine." Participants described this term to mean when a person shares information without any personal or financial gain. A Hispanic-Black female used this word when judging the authenticity of information:

> *I believe that having someone that's genuine, but you know, America runs on money. If there's someone that is not looking for what exactly they're gonna give me, even if it's not going to benefit you in a financial way, giving information that is factual. Everyone, everyone is different. Everyone's body is different. So, if your answer for every single person is oh, you should get the vaccine, then it's not really going to be something that's easily believable. You should be able to also be like, "Oh, you know, based on your health, based on what you have going on in your life, this is what I would advise." And it'd be different information that follows along with different people, because people's bodies are different. People's bodies react differently to different things. And just again, yeah, seeing someone that's not in it for what they're going to financially gain from, from what they're advising.*

Another participant, identifying as a Black Hispanic female, stated:

> *There hasn't been any differentiation, you know, between the ones who are vaccinated and those who aren't. So, there's no current, there's no current push to get it if someone's still going to get sick, or if it's still going to be able to be spread. There's no real reason, that I see personally, to get it.*

Another participant who identified as a Black Hispanic female felt unnaturally forced, raising her suspicions of the motives for mandatory vaccination.

> *If there's legitimate information that is put out through a reputable source, explaining, not just trying to, like force people to take a vaccine because there was a lot of that going on where it was like, "take the vaccine, you're gonna have to take it, you can't go anywhere if you don't, or you're not able to travel." It just seems kind of odd for anything, because I don't think there's been anything that's been treated like that. Especially not here in America, where it's like, oh, you're, you're gonna have certain rights taken away, if you don't.*

There were mixed responses of participant perceptions of COVID-19 information quality in the community. Responses encompassed all forms of COVID-19 information they encountered (e.g., news and social media) and not just information they received from health providers or the community.

Some participants felt they received quality information about COVID-19 that was detailed enough to make an informed decision about their health. Others noted conflicting information from untrustworthy sources. A few indicated that the information improved over time and was easy to understand. One non-Hispanic Black female said:

> *It's gotten a whole lot better. We've been at this for a good minute. The information as far as I'm concerned, is better, is more practical. [...] They make it plain so that I feel that you can understand it.*

In conclusion, there were overall feelings that COVID-19 information early in the pandemic was confusing and inconsistent. The knowledge was changing rapidly as more information was learned about infectivity, susceptibility, symptoms, and the vaccine. Information was received from various sources, including word of mouth, the internet and social media, and news on television and radio. There were concerns that the information from different sources was not unified and often contradicted each other. Participants were concerned about quality and verifiable information from sources and frequently did not know what information to believe. Trusted sources of information included local health providers, hospitals, and local government, especially if they knew individuals who worked in those fields [11].

Many participants were still not vaccinated at the time of the focus groups. Table 9.1 outlines the reasons participants did not get vaccinated. There were overall feelings of vaccine hesitancy due partly to safety concerns and the speed at which the clinical trials were completed with the vaccine subsequently approved for release. They perceived that information in the community about vaccines was good quality but still decided not to get vaccinated. Many were waiting for more information about long-term side effects or wanted alternative options to the vaccine. Many participants believed in homeopathic and non-westernized medicine methods and frequently cited herbalism for prevention and treatments.

Participants trusted health providers but shared that their doctors did not always initiate conversations about or encourage them to take the vaccine. Instead, they felt they could ask questions if they needed to. Other impactful messages came from reports of deaths and COVID-19 illness experiences, both in the news and among family and friends.

Table 9.1 Reasons for not receiving the COVID-19 vaccine [11]

Reasons	N	Percentage
I am concerned about the safety of the COVID-19 vaccines	60	25.32%
I do not think getting COVID-19 is a big threat to my health	16	6.75%
I do not think the COVID-19 vaccine will protect me from COVID-19	33	13.92%
My family members do not want me to get the COVID-19 vaccine	23	9.70%
I do not know where to get a COVID-19 vaccine	17	7.17%
The places to get a COVID-19 vaccine are not open during the times I need	8	3.38%
I have a medical condition that makes me unable to get the COVID-19 vaccine	14	5.91%
I have a religious or cultural reason that makes me unable to get the COVID-19 vaccine	30	12.66%
I have no particular reason why I have not received a COVID-19 vaccine	36	15.19%

Participants gave valuable feedback on how to improve COVID-19 information in the future. This included concise, unified messages from respected sources such as health professionals and local government. The information should consist of a unified message about COVID-19 and information about overall personal protections and infection control for healthy lifestyles (e.g., hand hygiene) so that the community is better prepared for future outbreaks. Participants still anticipate answers to questions regarding the origin of COVID-19, the long-term effects of the disease on physical and mental health, and the potential adverse effects of the COVID-19 vaccine. Participants emphasized cultural and age-appropriate education, consideration, and respect for all lifestyles and personal choices, including those who practice holistic and herbal medicine and those who believe in a Higher Power or prayer for protection from illness and death. Participants shared and discussed the information with family, friends, and community members, especially if they felt that the information came from a qualified source.

Suggestions on how the community could be reached varied by age and written or spoken communication preferences. Participants valued written, quality information to refer to it for confirmation, clarification, or verification from other sources. Other participants valued in-person (preferred) or virtual interpersonal communication so that questions could be answered. Information should be in places where people naturally gather, such as community events, supermarkets, and churches, but also available on local news, radio, the internet, and other forms of media so that maximum reach is achieved [11].

9.4 Cultural Humility and Social Determinants of Health

Early in our team's work with our diverse South Florida community, it became evident that there was a striking lack of health education materials that reflected our richly diverse community's visual, linguistic, and cultural preferences. Moreover, race and ethnicity categories did not give comprehensive options for our Caribbean community members to identify themselves adequately. This rendered the community effectively invisible. This partially explains the dearth of research and data on the Caribbean diaspora as a population of focus [12].

When specifically looking at vaccine hesitancy in communities of color, it is vital for clinicians to look inward—addressing assumptions/biases, understanding power structures and privilege, embracing how your lived experience impacts your interaction, and engaging in positive evolution through reflective practice. Employing a culturally humble approach focuses on patients as individuals—lending respect to unique components affecting each patient's decision-making lens.

In addition to looking inward, it is imperative to look outward—amplifying and addressing the voices and needs of the patients we treat, considering health equity in the context of intersectionality, developing and nurturing supportive patient-centered partnerships, and working together to dismantle and change privilege and power systems that contribute to adverse patient outcomes. As physicians, we are

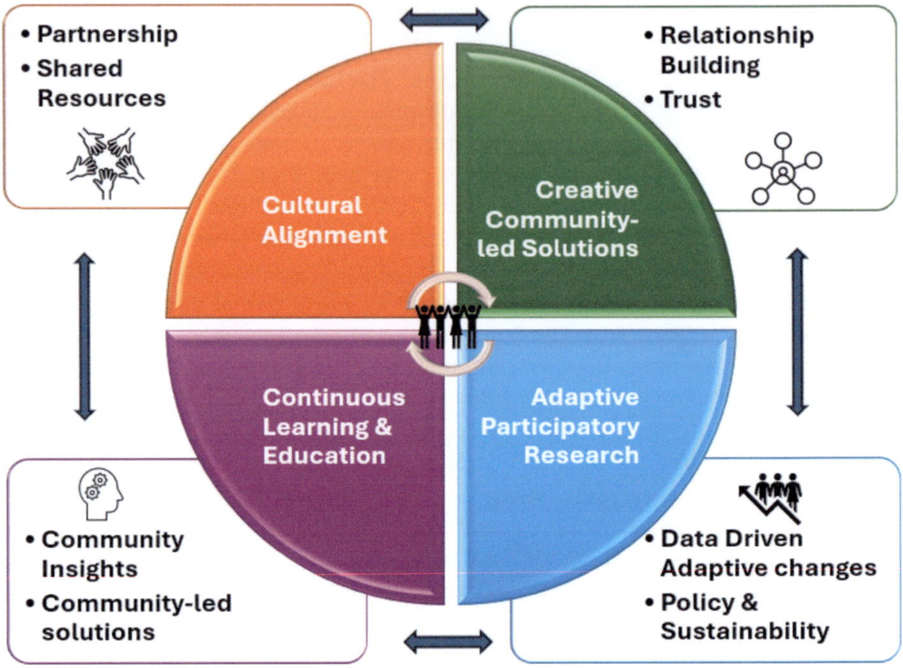

Fig. 9.1 Collaborative health equity research model

responsible to those we serve in a greater capacity than just the clinical care encounter. This includes addressing social determinants of health, actively advocating for structural and institutional change, and refining our approach to patient care to ensure we meet our patients' needs. Figure 9.1 illustrates the research model we used in our health equity initiatives. Our community- and person-centered approach is a continuous, dynamic process driven by community insights and creative data collection models through partnerships anchored in building trust and sharing resources.

Social determinants of health (SDOH), as outlined in Fig. 9.2, contribute significantly to overall health and wellness. This includes access to vaccines and social, psychological, and environmental conditions supporting an individual's overall well-being. The Office of Disease Prevention and Health Promotion defines the social determinants of health as "the conditions in the environments where people are born, live, learn, work, play, worship, and age that affect a wide range of health, functioning, and quality-of-life outcomes and risks" and groups them into five areas:

- Education access and quality
- Economic stability
- Social and community context
- Neighborhood and built environment
- Healthcare access and quality [13]

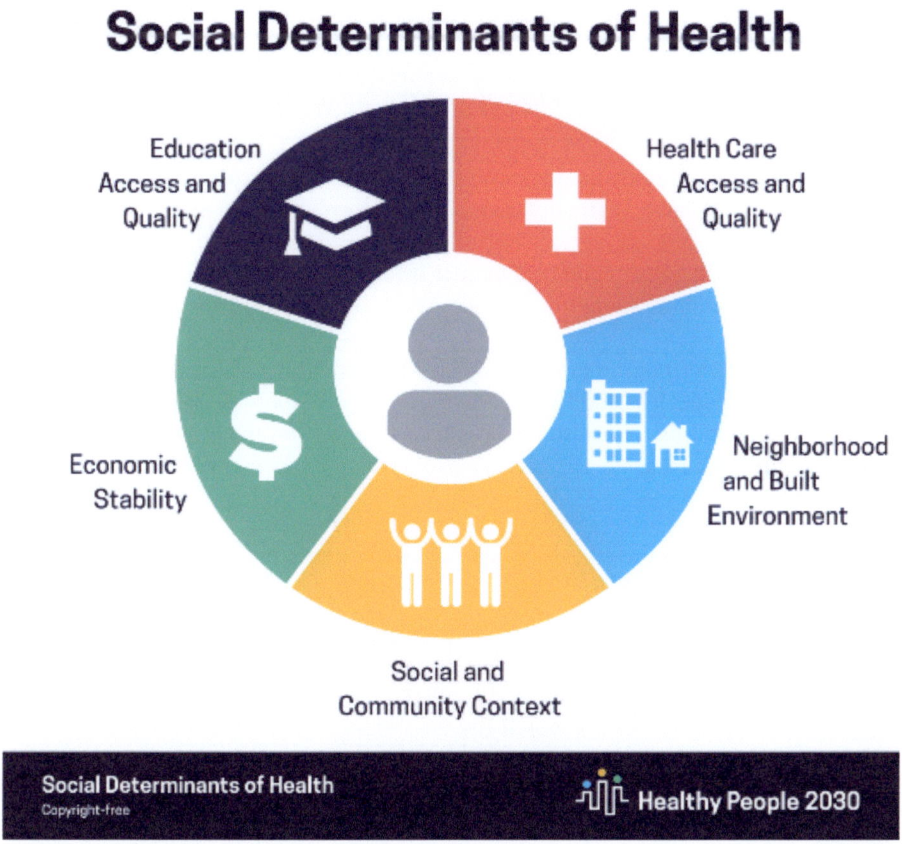

Fig. 9.2 Healthy People 2030, U.S. Department of Health and Human Services, Office of Disease Prevention and Health Promotion. (Retrieved May 1st, 2024, from https://health.gov/healthypeople/objectives-and-data/social-determinants-health [26])

Patients come from a variety of backgrounds and lived experiences. Capturing SDOH details is integral to better understanding our patients' decision-making lens. Capturing this data through electronic medical record surveys or partnering with community and other healthcare organizations to garner these details are viable solutions. Using smart features of Electronic Health Record (EHR) check-in systems allows patients to complete SDOH surveys at a convenient time/place before their office visit. In addition, creating an efficient yet dynamic healthcare team to ensure these vital details are retrieved in a manner that respects a patient's culture, language, reading readiness, and privacy is crucial. Using the SDOH framework, below is a list of granular areas that may impact vaccination:

9.4.1 Education Access and Quality

This multidimensional domain encompasses health literacy, language, and level of education. Examples include:

- People with a limited understanding of medical jargon or vaccine education materials may have difficulty using the information to make an informed decision.
- Difficulty identifying reputable, factual information through multiple information sources such as social media, television, online platforms, radio, and other sources.
- People from low-income families, those with disabilities, and those who experience bullying are less likely to perform well in school—negatively impacting their understanding of health information. In addition, the quality of education received plays a role.

9.4.2 Economic Stability

According to Ross and Dorazio in their publication "The Latest Poverty, Income, and Food Insecurity Data Reveal Continuing Racial Disparities," economic disparities persist in the United States, and the official poverty measure (OPM) includes annual pre-tax income from sources such as social security, income and unemployment. The supplemental poverty measure (SPM) takes into account factors such as housing, food, and tax benefits, as well as childcare and geographic differences. Figure 9.3 shows persistent disparities in poverty rates in 2023 [14, 31].

9.4.3 Economic Instability Can Impact Vaccine Hesitancy in the Following Ways

- Perceived costs of vaccinations and the impact of those financial commitments on daily life.
- High cost of healthcare, housing, and eating healthy foods causes reprioritizing of life tasks to ensure basic needs are met.
- The high cost of managing chronic, complicated medical conditions may supersede the need to think about vaccination.
- Concerns that vaccine adverse effects may negatively impact a person's ability to work or have a viable income source.
- On the other hand, vaccination may be viewed as a way to ensure a person stays healthy enough to work and have a sustainable source of income. One study showed that messages highlighting economic and personal financial risk could increase the likelihood of a person deciding to get vaccinated [15].

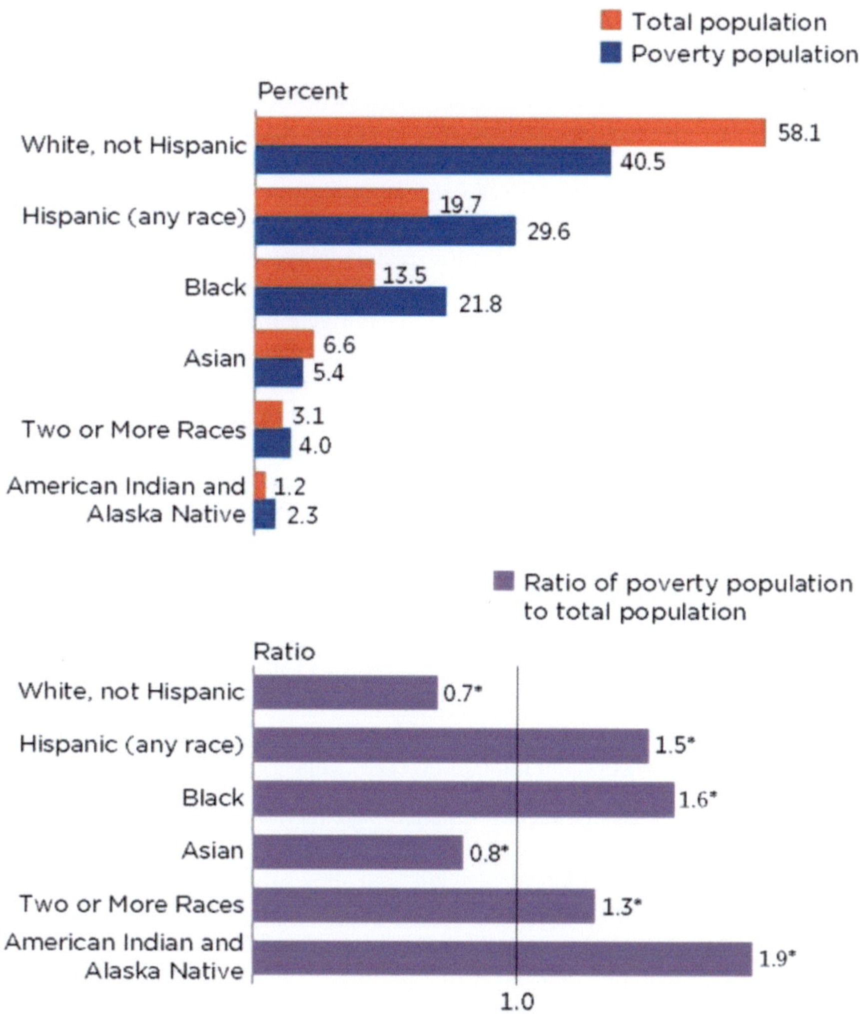

* An asterisk denotes that the ratio is different from 1.0 at the 90 percent confidence level.
Note: Population as of March of the following year. Information on confidentiality protection, sampling error, nonsampling error, and definitions is available at <https://www2.census.gov/programs-surveys/cps/techdocs/cpsmar24.pdf>.
Source: U.S. Census Bureau, Current Population Survey, 2024 Annual Social and Economic Supplement (CPS ASEC).

Fig. 9.3 Shrider, E. Distribution of total population and poverty by race and Hispanic origin using the official poverty measure: 2023 [31]

9.4.4 Social and Community Context

This SDOH domain is anchored by social circumstance, interpersonal interactions/influence, communication, cultural and religious beliefs, and trust. Vaccination decisions can be viewed socially as a declaration of one's relationships, political affinity, identity, and acceptance of community/family views [16]. Our research in predominantly Caribbean communities found that social structures, religious beliefs, family dynamics, and cultural factors played a large part in healthcare decision-making. Cultural factors included alternative "natural" treatments, holistic medicine, and prayer as ways to prevent or mitigate disease states. Western medicine often dismisses such practices as acceptable since a dearth of evidence-based research supports efficacy. This is an important area to explore as clinicians since respecting and acknowledging the concomitant use of culturally rooted measures alongside traditional medical recommendations can move the needle toward more trust and acceptance of clinical guidance.

In this domain, there is community engagement. It is imperative to engage communities in solid and lasting partnerships and to ensure solutions are co-created in ways that amplify and honor the needs and voices of those we seek to serve. One avenue to achieve these goals is through community-based participatory research that is dynamic, collaborative, and adaptive [17]. Figure 9.1 illustrates this model and aligns well with the team's approach. Our work with the City of Lauderhill residents is an example that reflects this research model. In addition, our team used the five-step collaboration cycle to anchor our work and build trust. This model translates well to patient–clinician interaction. The cycle consists of:

- Empathy—increases connection, patient satisfaction, and the likelihood of follow-up and engagement.
- Align motivation—evokes change talk and allows discovery of intrinsic motivators that drive health decisions.
- Build confidence—remind patients about successful ways they achieved past health goals and allow discovery of strengths.
- Set **SMART** goals—**S**pecific, **M**easurable, **A**ction-oriented/Achievable, **R**ealistic, and **T**ime-sensitive.
- Set accountability—arranging self-monitoring, buddy systems, and check-in with the patient.

This collaborative cycle pairs well with motivational interviewing to enhance the embrace and uptake of clinical recommendations [18]. Later in this chapter, I will expand my discussion on this five-step cycle and discuss motivational interviewing and a COACH approach in healthcare as successful strategies.

The National Academy of Medicine created a visual representation (Fig. 9.4) in their publication Assessing Meaningful Community Engagement: *A Conceptual Model to Advance Health Equity through Transformed Systems for Health* that summarizes salient components that support solid community engagement. According to the authors, "When health and healthcare policies and programs designed to

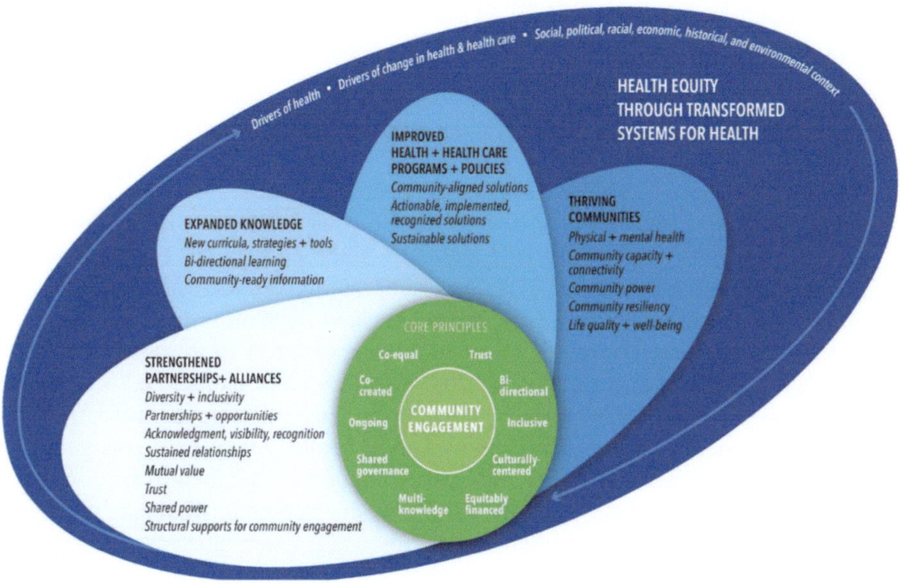

Fig. 9.4 Health Equity Through Transformed Systems For Health. Organizing Committee for Assessing Meaningful Community Engagement in Health & Health Care Programs & Policies. 2022. Assessing Meaningful Community Engagement: A Conceptual Model to Advance Health Equity through Transformed Systems for Health. NAM Perspectives. Commentary, National Academy of Medicine, Washington, DC. doi:10.31478/202202c. (Reproduced with permission from the National Academy of Sciences, Courtesy of the National Academies Press, Washington, D.C [19])

improve outcomes are not driven by community interests, concerns, assets, and needs, these efforts remain disconnected from the people they intend to serve. This disconnect ultimately limits the influence and effectiveness of interventions, policies, and programs" [19].

9.4.5 Neighborhood and Built Environment

This SDOH domain is also multidimensional and includes spaces where people live, work, play, eat, worship, and age. This domain has a massive impact on population health and individual decision-making. The complex interplay of elements that comprise the lived environment plays a substantial role in an individual's health, prioritization of needs/wants, and healthcare decisions such as vaccination. Story et al. generated an ecological framework to describe factors influencing what people eat. These variables are also intimately tied to a decision to receive vaccination. This framework captures the complexity and interplay of determinants that range from individual to societal aspects co-existing in a dynamic state, ultimately influencing the health and healthcare decisions of individuals [20]. The following examples highlight some of these variables impacting vaccination:

- Physical Infrastructure: The built environment determines access to healthcare and other vaccination facilities. Public transportation and walkable neighborhoods also affect access.
- Social Networks: An individual's family, peers, and trusted individuals such as religious leaders and primary care physicians can influence vaccination decisions. In our study in the City of Lauderhill, some participants only decided to get vaccinated against COVID-19 after seeing family members and close friends afflicted with complications or after being asked by family, friends, and their primary care physicians to get vaccinated. The proximity of these social circles to vaccine access may also play a role in vaccination decisions.
- Environmental Safety, Work, and Education: This sub-domain impacts well-being, informed decision-making, and overall health. Many participants in our study worked long hours at distant locations that prevented them from accessing vaccines. In addition, if a work or community environment is not safe or crime-ridden, an individual is less likely to consider vaccination since they focus time and energy on safety with ongoing vigilance. Moreover, easy access to culturally tailored and co-created vaccination education materials plays a major role in contemplating and eventually getting vaccinated. Ideally, these educational materials should incorporate evidence-based behavior change models such as the Health Belief model in structuring these educational resources to suit the media of choice (social media, radio, print, dialogue, etc.) [17].

9.4.6 Healthcare Access and Quality

As the topic title describes, access to, affordability, and availability of quality healthcare are integral to overall health and well-being. Case managers, community health workers, and social workers can assist as patient navigators to address each area. All members of an interprofessional healthcare team are touchpoints for patients, and all help to shape patients' trust, confidence in the health system, and ease of use. In the advancing age of technology, where artificial intelligence (AI) can take over rote tasks, we may finally have an opportunity to truly bring back the humanistic side of medicine. Face-to-face, meaningful, engaging, personal interactions are critical elements of patient-centered medicine. These are also tied to organizational, institutional, and other policies that govern or set guard rails and guidance for healthcare teams. It is imperative that we use technology to understand the intersectionality and unique SDOH impacting each patient. Emerging AI technologies may help restore joy in medical practice, which can translate to better patient outcomes, which include vaccination that protects against a host of preventable infections.

The clinical care experience must be positive to nurture trust and allow patients to feel connected enough to their clinical team to share their thoughts and concerns about vaccination. This nonjudgmental interaction should create a safe space for meaningful discussion. Clinicians face many administrative burdens and time limitations that can negatively impact longitudinal trust and relationship-building with patients. In addition, the inefficiencies and multilevel complexity that burden healthcare systems make it difficult or near impossible for patients to navigate it. In our City of Lauderhill COVID-19 health literacy and vaccination study, many participants voiced that their physicians and healthcare providers rarely initiated conversations about vaccines. It's important to recognize that the pandemic was an exceptionally challenging time for clinicians. This added to physician burnout, ultimately compromising patient care. Despite these frustrations, we must honor our patients' wishes to have these important issues addressed by the healthcare team.

9.5 Communication Strategies for Addressing Vaccine Hesitancy

Effective, collaborative patient–clinician communication is another important pillar in this SDOH domain. The **COACH** (**C**uriosity, **O**pen, **A**ppreciative, **C**ompassionate, **H**onesty) approach paired with motivational interviewing has the strongest chance of success in addressing vaccine hesitancy, apathy, or resistance. The COACH approach is a collaborative, supportive, and empowering form of interaction that can move the needle toward evidence-based health decision-making in patients of all cultures and backgrounds. In contrast, the **EXPERT** (**E**xamine, **X**-ray/diagnostics, **P**lan, **E**xplain, **R**ecommend, **T**ell, and sell) approach works best in acute care settings when patients require quick, life-saving interventions. In this latter approach, there is no time for collaboration and co-creation of action plans [21]. Pairing this COACH approach with motivational interviewing and the five-step collaboration cycle is a powerful combination that nurtures and fortifies trust, empowers patients to co-create actionable plans, and allows for exploring creative solutions that impact vaccination decisions. This includes patients taking an active role in their community and local government events, projects, and initiatives as health advocates to address SDOH that impact their lives and resources. We took a similar approach in our health literacy and health equity research by ensuring our community-based participatory research model honored the voices and choices of the community we served [11, 12, 18, 22]. Here are the five steps of the Collaboration Cycle:

1. Empathy
2. Aligning motivation
3. Building confidence
4. Setting **SMART** goals (**S**pecific, **M**easurable, **A**ction Oriented/**A**chievable, **R**elevant, and **T**ime-based)
5. Accountability

9.5.1 Empathy

Studies show that genuine caring and sensitive kindness increase patient happiness, engagement, trust, connection, and likelihood of follow-up. Our choice of words, tone, and body language are all tied to expressing empathy. This also includes being nonjudgmental, respectful, and genuinely listening to our patients, understanding the unique yet complex, dynamic layers of intersectional lived experiences that constitute each individual. In today's fast-moving healthcare environment, slowing down just enough to truly "connect" with our patients is challenging. As noted earlier, I hope that artificial intelligence, if synergistically, ethically, and productively aligned in healthcare infrastructure, will allow us as clinicians to be more human with our patients and allow our empathy and compassion to grow and thrive. Bringing this joy back into medicine has a positive ripple effect on patient care and outcomes.

9.5.2 Aligning Motivation

In this part of the cycle, we are seeking to explore a patient's intrinsic motivations for decisions such as not getting vaccinated. Employing open-ended, nonjudgmental questions can bring this to light. For a patient who is not vaccinated, here are some questions you can ask: *Why is not getting vaccinated important to you? Are there any specific concerns you have about getting vaccinated?* One of the goals here is to discover personal motivations and address them in a kind, considerate manner. This empowers patients to become change agents in their own care. Helping patients discover their internal motivations allows them to become powerful architects of their circumstances, health, and well-being.

9.5.3 Building Confidence

This part of the cycle involves unearthing a patient's strengths and past successes through a motivational interviewing process. Drawing parallels to similar situations with positive outcomes allows for the precipitation of confidence and empowerment to overcome challenges and find creative ways to make healthy decisions.

9.5.4 Setting SMART Goals and Being Accountable

At this last stage of the cycle, you are setting **S**pecific, **M**easurable, **A**ction-oriented (or **A**chievable), **R**ealistic, and **T**ime-sensitive goals that keep you accountable. All these components are necessary for these steps to be effective. A clear example a patient can commit to is: "I want to come back in 3 months to your office to get vaccinated for the first time. I will come during my time off from work as your last evening appointment." Here is an analysis of this statement that shows it is a SMART goal:

Specific—getting vaccinated in 3 months.
Measurable—coming back to the office to get vaccinated.
Action-oriented/Achievable—taking the initiative to schedule an appointment and return to the office.
Realistic—choosing an appointment slot that aligns well with time off from work.
Time-sensitive— within a 3-month time frame, choosing the last appointment and ensuring a time to return to the office for vaccination and discussion.

Communication, as the spoken word, also includes educational resources/interventions through various formats, such as digital, printed, face-to-face, social media, and other ways, and should incorporate culturally appropriate behavior change theories as a framework to construct and deliver actionable health messaging. Behavior change theories such as the Health Belief Model (HBM) can allow clinicians to gain a deeper understanding of the intersectionality of individuals—how lived experiences and a multilayered complex mix of elements play a role in behavior change, such as embracing vaccination. According to Li et al., "The HBM posits four principal drivers of health behaviors: people's knowledge and perception of the severity of disease and their susceptibility to it; people's perception of the barriers to and benefits of being vaccinated; self-efficacy, that is, their belief in their ability to be vaccinated; and the cues to action." In addition, fostering trust through transparency, co-creation of health messaging, and cultural humility is vital in making positive behavioral changes. Studies show that behavioral theory-based interventions had more measurability and effectiveness in positive behavior change [23].

Pierz et al. in their article, "Supporting US Healthcare Providers for Successful Vaccine Communication," describe the following insightful findings:

> *44 focus group participants representing 24 US states with the majority (80%) fully vaccinated at the time of data collection. Most participants were doctors (34%) or physician's assistants and nurse practitioners (34%). The negative impact of COVID-19 misinformation on patient-provider communication at both intrapersonal and interpersonal levels as well as barriers and facilitators to patient vaccine uptake are reported. People or sources that play a role in health communication ("messengers") and persuasive messages that impact behavior or attitudes towards vaccination ("messages") are described. Providers expressed frustration in the need to continuously address vaccine misinformation in clinical appointments among patients who remained unvaccinated. Many providers found value in resources that provided up-to-date and evidence-based information as COVID-19 guidelines continued to change. Additionally, providers indicated that patient-facing materials designed to support vaccination education were not frequently available, but they were the most valuable to providers in a changing information environment* [24].

Ensuring that culturally appropriate, actionable vaccine education resources are available in a language and format preferred by patients is ideal. Moreover, "who" is delivering health messaging is just as important, or sometimes more important, in determining vaccination decisions. If a patient–clinician dyad is already rooted in trust or perhaps there is cultural common ground that allows open expression of alternative or holistic options that can pair nicely with evidence-based vaccine recommendations without causing harm—there is a great chance for success in vaccination decisions. In my experience working with culturally diverse communities, this approach was very effective. For example, if a patient prefers using herbs and special prayers as an adjunct to vaccination, clinicians should embrace it! This may go against traditional medical training, but it also honors and respects a patient's preferences if the alternative options discussed are safe and cause no harm.

The quality of healthcare services is also within this SDOH domain. This refers to access to evidence-based recommendations and staff competency, professionalism, empathy, compassion, and transparency. In addition, cultural humility and language access are essential pillars of this dynamic interaction. According to the CDC's Global Public Health Equity Guiding Principles for Communication:

> Cultural humility *is active engagement in an ongoing process of self-reflection, in which individuals seek to:*
>
> - *Examine their personal history/background and social position related to gender, ethnicity, socioeconomic status, profession, education, assumptions, values, beliefs, biases, and culture, and how these factors impact interpersonal interactions.*
> - *Reflect on how interpersonal interactions and relationships are impacted by the history, biases, norms, perception, and relative position of power of one's professional organization.*
> - *Gain deeper realization, understanding, and respect of cultural differences through active inquiry, reflection, reflexivity, openness to establishing power-balanced relationships, and appreciation of another person's/community's/population's expertise on the social and cultural context of their own lives (lived experience) and contributions to public health and wellbeing.*
> - *Recognize areas in which they do not have all the relevant experience and expertise and demonstrate a nonjudgmental willingness to learn from a person/community/population about their experiences and practices* [25].

9.6 Conclusion and Recommendations

In this section, I expound on various communication channels and strategies that support a decision to get vaccinated in SDOH-based communication venues: healthcare facilities, schools, work, government (local, state, national), community initiatives, and partnerships.

All areas, venues, and touchpoints where people work, live, eat, play, worship, and age are opportunities for engagement and culturally, patient-centric information sharing. Messaging and calls to action should be delivered by trusted community members from eclectic backgrounds such as healthcare, religion, or within a circle of influence for each patient. Behavioral theory-based interventions tailored to the type of interaction (e.g., social media, face-to-face, open community dialogue) have been shown to be most effective in facilitating positive behavior change.

Transparent, inclusive, and personalized vaccination initiatives that are science-supported should be woven into all forms of communication and not limited to healthcare personnel and institutions. In our research in the City of Lauderhill, we found a significant number of our participants obtained vaccine safety information from their barbers, places of worship, community business owners, and other non-health entities. Ensuring people involved in information delivery are using scientifically backed details is imperative. This also helps to get ahead of misinformation and dispel any myths. One way to achieve this is to create an easily accessible and adaptive education training curriculum for community members.

Community influencers are powerful agents of information dissemination and acceptance. This power can be harnessed to ensure factual information is shared with community members who may be in a contemplation state, planting the seeds of thought toward positive health decisions. Ultimately, a person's circumstance and intersection of relevant SDOH are dynamic and ever-changing. Leaning on the COACH approach and tapping into our emotional intelligence and cultural awareness creates a safe space to build trust and facilitate positive patient outcomes.

Building a fluid, adaptive, and synergistic communication system that acts in concert with the unique needs of our community allows for overall success in public health necessities such as vaccination. This involves collaborating and co-creating creative strategies and systems at national, state, local, community, and individual levels. A critical review of lessons learned from the COVID-19 pandemic and the evolving body of data that highlights successes and failures can be used to refine our approach. Addressing vaccine hesitancy requires us to take a meaningful look at how our past shapes our present. Contemporary issues such as biases, structural racism, disparities in underserved and vulnerable communities, and lack of adequate culturally tailored resources must be addressed for us to achieve health equity. The CDC's Vaccination Field Guide summarizes key areas of focus such as [28]:

- Vaccine ambassadors
- Home, school, and work delivered vaccinations
- Financial incentives
- Provider recommendation and standardization support
- Trustworthy messaging and reminders

The following additional resources described in Table 9.2 can be used to address vaccination challenges and augment our collective abilities to keep our community healthy, well, and protected from preventable diseases.

Table 9.2 Additional resources to address vaccine hesitancy in diverse communities

Resource type	Weblink
Chapter focused on cultural competency and vaccine hesitancy [29]	https://www.immunizationmanagers.org/content/uploads/2022/03/Vaccine-Confidence-Guide-Chapter-2_033022.pdf
Vaccine confidence tool kits [30]	https://www.acpm.org/initiatives/power-of-prevention/vaccine-confident/#toolkit
CDC vaccine confidence strategy [28]	https://www.cdc.gov/vaccines/partners/vaccinate-with-confidence.html
Increasing vaccination through psychological science [2, 3]	https://pubmed.ncbi.nlm.nih.gov/29611455/
CDC community field guide strategies [27]	https://www.cdc.gov/vaccines/covid-19/downloads/vaccination-strategies.pdf

References

1. MacDonald NE. Vaccine hesitancy: definition, scope and determinants. Vaccine. 2015;33(34):4161–4. https://doi.org/10.1016/j.vaccine.2015.04.036.
2. Brewer NT, et al. Increasing vaccination: putting psychological science into action. Psychol Sci Public Interest. 2017;18(1):149–207. https://doi.org/10.1177/1529100618760521.
3. Abad N, Messinger S, Huang Q, Hendrich M. A qualitative study of behavioral and social drivers of COVID-19 vaccine confidence and uptake among unvaccinated Americans in the US April–May 2021. PLoS One. 2023;18(2):e0281497.
4. Centers for Disease Control and Prevention. (n.d.). The Untreated Syphilis Study at Tuskegee Timeline. Retrieved May 1, 2024, from https://www.cdc.gov/tuskegee/timeline.htm
5. Holland B. The 'father of modern gynecology' performed shocking experiments on enslaved women. HISTORY; 2017, August 29. Retrieved April 22, 2024, from https://www.history.com/news/the-father-of-modern-gynecology-performed-shocking-experiments-on-slaves
6. Nuriddin A, et al. Reckoning with histories of medical racism and violence in the USA. Lancet. 2020;396(10256):949–51. https://doi.org/10.1016/S0140-6736(20)32032-8.
7. Newman PA, Dinh DA, Nyoni T, et al. Covid-19 vaccine hesitancy and under-vaccination among marginalized populations in the United States and Canada: a scoping review. J Racial Ethn Health Disparities. 2023;12:413. https://doi.org/10.1007/s40615-023-01882-1.
8. Willis DE, et al. COVID-19 vaccine hesitancy and racial discrimination among US adults. Prev Med Rep. 2022;31:102074. https://doi.org/10.1016/j.pmedr.2022.102074.
9. Savoia E, Piltch-Loeb R, Goldberg B, Miller-Idriss C, Hughes B, Montrond AM, Kayyem JN, Testa MA. Predictors of COVID-19 vaccine hesitancy: socio-demographics, co-morbidity and past experience of racial discrimination. medRxiv. 2021; https://doi.org/10.1101/2021.01.12.21249152.
10. Siegel M, Critchfield-Jain I, Boykin M, Owens A, Muratore R, Nunn T, Oh J. Racial/ethnic disparities in state-level COVID-19 vaccination rates and their association with structural racism. J Racial Ethn Health Disparities. 2022;9(6):2361–74. https://doi.org/10.1007/s40615-021-01173-7.
11. Haffizulla F, Hollar L, Alamu J, Biggs E, Navarro C, Montoya M, Andzenge A, Wall A, Mullings B, Ownby R. Advancing health literacy to enhance equitable community responses to COVID-19—Grant report. Retrieved from NSU Teams Database: AHL HHS NSU Internal; 2023.
12. Haffizulla FS, et al. Caribbean diaspora healthy nutrition outreach project (CDHNOP): a qualitative and quantitative approach to Caribbean health. Ann Glob Health. 2020;86(1):12. https://doi.org/10.5334/aogh.2657.
13. Yelton B, Friedman D, Friedman D, Noblet S, Lohman M, Arent M, Macauda M, Sakhuja M, Leith K. Social determinants of health and depression among African American adults: a scoping review of current research. Int J Environ Res Public Health. 2022;19(3):1498.
14. Ross K, Dorazio J. The latest poverty, income and food insecurity data reveal continuing racial disparities. Center for American Progress; 2022, December 21. Retrieved May 1, 2024, from https://www.americanprogress.org/article/the-latest-poverty-income-and-food-insecurity-data-reveal-continuing-racial-disparities/
15. Zhong W, Broniatowski DA. Economic risk framing increases intention to vaccinate among republican COVID-19 vaccine refusers. Soc Sci Med. 2023;317:115594. https://doi.org/10.1016/j.socscimed.2022.115594.
16. Milionis C, Ilias I, Tselebis A, Pachi A. Psychological and social aspects of vaccination hesitancy-implications for travel medicine in the aftermath of the COVID-19 crisis: a narrative review. Medicina (Kaunas). 2023;59(10):1744. https://doi.org/10.3390/medicina59101744.
17. Chanita Hughes Halbert. Caitlin G Allen, basic behavioral science research priorities in minority health and health disparities, translational. Behav Med. 2021;11(11):2033–42. https://doi.org/10.1093/tbm/ibab143.

18. Frates E. The five step collaboration cycle: a tool for the doctor's office. IJSCP. 2015;2:1–5. https://doi.org/10.4172/ijscp.1000144.
19. Organizing Committee for Assessing Meaningful Community Engagement in Health & Health Care Programs & Policies. Assessing Meaningful Community Engagement: a conceptual model to advance health equity through transformed systems for health. NAM Perspectives. Commentary, National Academy of Medicine, Washington, DC; 2022. https://doi.org/10.31478/202202c.
20. Story M, Kaphingst KM, Robinson-O'Brien R, Glanz K. Creating healthy food and eating environments: policy and environmental approaches. Annu Rev Public Health. 2008;29:253–72. https://doi.org/10.1146/annurev.publhealth.29.020907.090926.
21. Moon M. Why the "coach approach" beats the expert approach for health coaches. Primal Health Coach Institute; 2021, May 18. Retrieved May 6, 2024, from https://www.primalhealthcoach.com/blog/why-the-coach-approach-beats-the-expert-approach-for-health-coaches/
22. City of Lauderhill Florida. (n.d.). Community needs assessment. Retrieved May 6, 2024, from https://online.fliphtml5.com/vuemf/edrq/
23. Li L, Wood CE, Kostkova P. Vaccine hesitancy and behavior change theory-based social media interventions: a systematic review. Transl Behav Med. 2022;12(2):243–72. https://doi.org/10.1093/tbm/ibab148.
24. Pierz AJ, Rauh L, Masoud D, Cruz AK, Palmedo PC, Ratzan SC, Parker R. Supporting US healthcare providers for successful vaccine communication. BMC Health Serv Res. 2023;23(1):423. https://doi.org/10.1186/s12913-023-09348-0.
25. Centers for Disease Control and Prevention. (n.d.). Global Health Equity. Principle 1: Embrace cultural humility and community engagement. Retrieved May 3, 2024, from https://www.cdc.gov/globalhealth/equity/guide/cultural-humility.html#print
26. Healthy People 2030, U.S. Department of Health and Human Services, Office of Disease Prevention and Health Promotion. (n.d.). Retrieved May 1, 2024, from https://health.gov/healthypeople/objectives-and-data/social-determinants-health
27. Centers for Disease Control and Prevention. COVID-19 Vaccination Field Guide: 12 Strategies for Your Community. Retrieved May 7th, 2024 from https://www.cdc.gov/vaccines/covid-19/downloads/vaccination-strategies.pdf
28. Centers for Disease Control and Prevention. COVID-19 Vaccination Field Guide: 12 Strategies for Your Community. Retrieved October 6th, 2024 from https://www.cdc.gov/vaccines/partners/vaccinate-with-confidence.html
29. Association of Immunization Managers. Vaccine Confidence Tool Kit. Retrieved October 6th, 2024 from https://www.immunizationmanagers.org/resources-toolkits/vaccine-confidence-toolkit/
30. American College of Preventive Medicine. Vaccine Confidence Tool Kits. Retrieved October 6th from https://www.acpm.org/initiatives/power-of-prevention/vaccine-confident/#toolkit
31. Shrider E A. "Poverty in the United States: 2023." Census.Gov, United States Census Bureau, 3 Sept. 2024, www.census.gov/library/publications/2024/demo/p60-283.html

Chapter 10
Putting It All Together: Cases for the Vaccine Hesitancy Curriculum

Nyla Dil and Amanda J. Chase

10.1 Introduction

The cases in this chapter serve as a valuable resource for active-learning sessions, offering real-life clinical scenarios that foster rich discussions about the benefits of vaccination. By examining these cases—chickenpox, influenza pneumonia, whooping cough, measles, and polio—health professions learners can engage deeply with the material, enhancing their understanding of the clinical features, pathogenesis, and prevention of vaccine-preventable diseases. These scenarios underscore the crucial role of clinicians in effectively communicating vaccine benefits and addressing hesitancy, ultimately preparing learners to support informed decision-making in their future practice.

10.2 Case 1: Chickenpox

This case focuses on the clinical features, pathogenesis, and prevention of a vaccine-preventable viral infection. Clinicians play a fundamental role in communicating with patients about vaccines and are typically their patients' primary source for

N. Dil
Department of Medical Education, College of Medicine, University of Central Florida, Orlando, FL, USA
e-mail: Nyla.Dil@ucf.edu

A. J. Chase (✉)
Department of Medical Education, Dr. Kiran C. Patel College of Allopathic Medicine, Nova Southeastern University, Fort Lauderdale, FL, USA
e-mail: achase0@nova.edu

A. J. Chase et al. (eds.), *Vaccine Hesitancy Curriculum*,
https://doi.org/10.1007/978-3-031-88668-3_10

vaccine information. Therefore, understanding the benefits of vaccination is crucial for health professions learners. Some vaccine-hesitant individuals believe that there is little risk to becoming infected with a vaccine-preventable infection. In this case, the child becomes susceptible to a life-threatening secondary bacterial infection.

10.2.1 Case 1 Clinical Vignette

Kenneth Gibson, a 5-year-old male, presents to his pediatrician, Dr. Mette, with a fever and a pruritic, vesicular rash of 48 h duration. Mrs. Gibson indicates that Kenneth developed a sore throat and loss of appetite about 2–3 days ago and "won't stop scratching."

Physical Examination

Vitals: 37.8 °C (100 °F); HR 130; BP 92/56; RR 22; SpO_2 96% on room air.

General: Alert and irritable. Well nourished; in no acute distress.

HEENT: PERRL. White sclerae. Mild pharyngeal and tonsillar erythema without exudates. membranes (TMs) clear.

Neck: A few scattered, nontender lymph nodes are palpable in the anterior cervical chains.

Integument: Scattered erythematous macules, papules, vesicles, and pustules on the scalp, face, abdomen, arms, hands, chest, and back.

Dr. Mette informs Mrs. Gibson that Kenneth has chickenpox. Dr. Mette inquires with Mrs. Gibson about Kenneth's varicella-zoster virus (VZV) vaccination status, and Mrs. Gibson indicates that she is opposed to vaccinations for health safety concerns. Neither Kenneth nor his two older brothers (ages 7 and 11) have received the VZV vaccine. Mrs. Gibson asks Dr. Mette about the likelihood of other members of the family developing chickenpox. Dr. Mette describes the mode of VZV transmission and offers information on the benefits and risks of vaccination. She advises Mrs. Gibson to keep Kenneth out of school until all of his blisters have crusted over.

Five days later, Kenneth returns to the clinic with a recurrent fever and erythematous swelling of the left hand.

Physical Examination

Vitals: 39 °C (102.2 °F); HR 145; BP 88/52; RR 26; SpO_2 96% on room air.

General: Crying and irritable.

HEENT: PERRL. White sclerae. No pharyngeal or tonsillar erythema. TMs clear.

Neck: No lymphadenopathy.

Integument: Diffusely, scattered crusted vesicles. Left hand, dorsum: honey-colored, crusted vesicles with an erythematous base and swelling, without streaking.

Extremities: Left epitrochlear lymph nodes are palpable.

Dr. Mette diagnoses Kenneth with cellulitis and admits him to the hospital. A CBC with differential and wound cultures are ordered. A scraping from the base of one of the lesions on the left hand is taken and two smear slides are stained with Gram stain and Wright stain, respectively. The Wright stain shows numerous neutrophils with scattered monocytes, lymphocytes, and multinucleated giant cells. Gram stain reveals Gram-positive cocci in chains. The peripheral white blood cell count is 16,000/mm^3 (reference = 4000–10,000/mm^3) with 90% neutrophils (reference = 40–80%).

Kenneth is diagnosed with streptococcal cellulitis of the left hand, due to *Streptococcus pyogenes*, secondary to traumatic excoriation of VZV blisters. Kenneth receives oxacillin IV with substantial improvement of the hand pain, erythema, and swelling noted overnight. The following morning, oxacillin IV is changed to PO amoxicillin, and Kenneth is discharged home.

Two days later, Dr. Mette phones Mrs. Gibson to inquire about Kenneth's status. Mrs. Gibson states that his hand has improved remarkably; however, she is concerned because her pregnant sister is coming to visit. She asks Dr. Mette if she should notify her sister to cancel her trip because of Kenneth's chickenpox; she adds that she and her siblings all had chickenpox when they were children. Dr. Mette states that her sister does not need to cancel her trip, but she does indicate that anyone with a history of chickenpox is susceptible to developing shingles as an adult.

10.2.2 Case 1 Learning Objectives

1. Recognize the importance of childhood vaccine risk/benefit communication.
2. Describe the clinical presentation and complications of chickenpox.
3. Describe the mode of transmission and course of infection of varicella-zoster virus.
4. Discuss the indications, contraindications, and formulation of the varicella vaccine.
5. Characterize the pathogenesis, diagnosis, and management of varicella-zoster virus.
6. Describe how Gram and Wright stains are used in the diagnosis of bacterial and viral infections.
7. Describe the clinical symptoms and treatment of cellulitis caused by *Streptococcus pyogenes*.
8. Characterize the clinical uses, mechanism of action, and antimicrobial spectrum of oxacillin and amoxicillin in addition to the development of resistance by target microbes.
9. Differentiate between chickenpox and shingles.

10.2.3 Case 1 Discussion

The multifaceted nature of vaccine hesitancy can make vaccine discussions with patients complex and highly charged. Following elicitation of the patient's or caregiver's chief concerns surrounding vaccination, the healthcare provider should accurately label their feeling and reflect its intensity. Next, the provider should discuss the benefits of vaccination and potential risks while avoiding medical jargon. The provider should check for understanding by asking the patient or caregiver to restate their understanding of the discussion. Finally, closure should be provided by briefly rephrasing the main points introduced in the discussion and seeking verification of understanding [1]. In this case, after the provider has the vaccine conversation with the mother, the mother's child is admitted to the hospital due to a dangerous bacterial infection of a chickenpox lesion. Learners should discuss the benefits of circling back to the vaccine conversation with the mother following the complication.

10.3 Case 2: Influenza Pneumonia

In this case, an unvaccinated patient presents with a severe case of influenza pneumonia. The patient is hospitalized as her condition worsens. Students will explore the characteristics of influenza virus infection, the immunological responses to viruses, and the concepts of antigenic shift and drift. Additionally, they will have the opportunity to discuss approaches to communication with vaccine-hesitant patients.

10.3.1 Case 2 Clinical Vignette

Katie Lorenzo is a 29-year-old female presenting to the Emergency Department with a 2-day history of fever, chills, headache, myalgia, cough, and dyspnea. Her symptoms began suddenly and are steadily getting worse. She has no significant past medical history, and she does not take routine medications. When asked if she received the annual influenza vaccine, Katie states that she doesn't believe in getting vaccinated because vaccines contain mercury. Review of systems is positive for fever, lethargy, shortness of breath, excessive sweating, and muscle soreness.

Physical Examination

Vitals: 39.6C (103.3 °F); HR 120; BP 120/76; RR 30; SpO_2 89% on room air, 94% on 2 L oxygen via nasal cannula.

General: Well nourished, diaphoretic, ill appearing with respiratory distress, tachypnea, and use of accessory muscles.

CV: Tachycardia without murmurs or rubs.

Lungs: Diffuse, bilateral wheezing and rales with diminished breath sounds at the bases.
Skin: Warm and moist.

Dr. Lee orders a chest X-ray, CBC with differential, sputum cultures, blood cultures, and a rapid antigen assay for influenza types A and B.

The chest radiograph reveals bilateral patchy interstitial infiltrates, most notably in the lung bases. Katie has an elevated white blood cell count of 11,400/mm^3 (reference = 3500–10,500/mm^3) with 87% segmented neutrophils and 9% lymphocytes. Rapid antigen assay of a nasal swab is positive for influenza A. Dr. Lee informs Katie that she likely has influenza pneumonia and explains that the influenza infection may be complicated by concomitant, or secondary bacterial pneumonia.

Katie is admitted to the hospital, started on oral oseltamivir, and continued on nasal oxygen. Dr. Lee performs the thoracic inhibitory pressure technique on the patient's upper thoracic region and myofascial release of the diaphragm. In addition, empiric IV antibiotics are initiated with bacterial blood culture results pending. As part of a local public health surveillance program, Dr. Lee sends a sputum sample to the local public health laboratory for confirmation and identification of influenza strain by RT-PCR.

Blood and sputum cultures for bacterial organisms are negative. Katie's SpO2 on room air normalizes and she is discharged on hospital day 3 to complete 5-day courses of oseltamivir and azithromycin. Subsequently, the public health laboratory reports molecular analysis of the sputum specimen to be positive for influenza A (H3N2).

10.3.2 Case 2 Learning Objectives

1. Describe the clinical presentation and management of influenza pneumonia.
2. Discuss the indications, contraindications, and formulation of the seasonal influenza vaccine.
3. Describe the pathophysiology of the immune response to influenza infections.
4. Evaluate the rationale for the administration of antibiotics following an influenza infection.
5. Describe the epidemiology, pathogenesis, and laboratory diagnosis of influenza A and B viruses.
6. Discuss the clinical uses and mechanism of action of oseltamivir in addition to the development of resistance.
7. Adopt a communication strategy that addresses patients' concerns about vaccine excipients.
8. Utilize metaphors to communicate the risks and benefits of vaccination with a patient.

10.3.3 Case 2 Discussion

The patient states that she does not receive any vaccines due to the belief that they all contain mercury. Thimerosal has been used in trace amounts in some vaccines since the 1930s to prevent bacterial and fungal contamination. It contains *ethyl mercury*, a form of organic mercury that does not accumulate in the body, unlike *methyl mercury*, a related form that does accumulate and is neurotoxic. Both forms of mercury occur naturally in the environment, in the air, soil, oceans, and in fish. Mercury is also used in various industrial processes, dental fillings, and thermometers. Mercury becomes harmful only when it reaches certain levels in the body, with toxicity depending on factors such as the amount and type of mercury consumed, body weight, and duration of exposure. Even though thimerosal use in medical products has a record of being very safe and data from many studies shows zero evidence of harm caused by the low doses of thimerosal in vaccines, thimerosal was taken out of childhood vaccines in the United States in 2001 [2, 3]. Metaphorical construction to communicate the importance of vaccination has been described [4] and metaphorical descriptions of the flu have been shown to increase people's expressed willingness to be vaccinated [5].

10.4 Case 3: Whooping Cough (Pertussis)

This case delves into the clinical features, pathogenesis, and prevention of whooping cough, a highly contagious bacterial infection caused by *Bordetella pertussis*. Whooping cough is a vaccine-preventable disease, yet it remains a significant public health concern, particularly among infants and young children who are not fully vaccinated. Clinicians play a fundamental role in educating patients and their families about the importance of vaccinations. They are often the primary source of vaccine information for their patients, making their role in promoting vaccine acceptance crucial.

Understanding the benefits of vaccination is essential for health professions learners, as they will encounter vaccine-hesitant individuals in their practice. These individuals may believe that the risks of vaccination outweigh the benefits or that there is little risk of contracting vaccine-preventable diseases. However, this case illustrates the severe consequences that can arise from such infections. In this scenario, a child who has not been vaccinated becomes susceptible to a life-threatening bacterial infection, highlighting the critical need for effective communication and education about vaccines.

10.4.1 Case 3 Clinical Vignette

James Carter, a 6-month-old male, presents to his pediatrician, Dr. Smith, with a severe cough that has persisted for two weeks. Mrs. Carter indicates that James has episodes of coughing that end with a high-pitched "whoop" sound and has been vomiting after coughing fits. He also has a runny nose and mild fever.

Physical Examination

Vitals: 38 °C (100.4 °F); HR 160; BP 85/45; RR 40; SpO2 94% on room air.
General: Alert but irritable. Well nourished; in no acute distress.
HEENT: PERRL. Mild nasal congestion. No pharyngeal erythema. TMs clear.
Neck: No lymphadenopathy.
Respiratory: Frequent coughing fits with inspiratory "whoop." Clear lung fields between coughing episodes.

Dr. Smith informs Mrs. Carter that James has whooping cough. Dr. Smith inquires with Mrs. Carter about James's DTaP (diphtheria, tetanus, and acellular pertussis) vaccination status, and Mrs. Carter indicates that she is opposed to vaccinations for health safety concerns. James has not received any doses of the DTaP vaccine. Mrs. Carter asks Dr. Smith about the likelihood of other members of the family developing whooping cough. Dr. Smith describes the mode of pertussis transmission and offers information on the benefits and risks of vaccination. She advises Mrs. Carter to keep James away from other children and to monitor for signs of respiratory distress.

Three days later, James returns to the clinic with increased difficulty breathing and cyanosis during coughing fits.

Physical Examination

Vitals: 39 °C (102.2 °F); HR 170; BP 80/40; RR 50; SpO2 88% on room air.
General: Crying and irritable.
HEENT: PERRL. Mild nasal congestion. No pharyngeal erythema. TMs clear.
Neck: No lymphadenopathy.
Respiratory: Frequent coughing fits with inspiratory "whoop." Diffuse crackles heard in both lung fields.

Dr. Smith diagnoses James with pertussis-associated pneumonia and admits him to the hospital. A CBC with differential and chest X-ray are ordered. The chest X-ray shows bilateral infiltrates consistent with pneumonia. The peripheral white blood cell count is 20,000/mm^3 (reference = 4000–10,000/mm^3) with 80% lymphocytes (reference = 20–40%).

James is diagnosed with bacterial pneumonia secondary to pertussis infection. He receives IV antibiotics and supportive care with substantial improvement in his respiratory symptoms noted overnight. The following morning, IV antibiotics are changed to oral antibiotics, and James is discharged home.

Two days later, Dr. Smith phones Mrs. Carter to inquire about James's status. Mrs. Carter states that James's breathing has improved remarkably; however, she is concerned because her elderly mother is coming to visit. She asks Dr. Smith if she should notify her mother to cancel her trip because of James's whooping cough. Dr. Smith states that her mother should avoid visiting until James has fully recovered, as pertussis can be particularly severe in older adults.

10.4.2 Case 3 Learning Objectives

1. Recognize the importance of effective communication about vaccine risks and benefits with caregivers.
2. Describe the clinical presentation and complications of whooping cough.
3. Explain the mode of transmission and course of infection of Bordetella pertussis.
4. Discuss the indications, contraindications, and formulation of the DTaP vaccine.
5. Characterize the pathogenesis, diagnosis, and management of pertussis.
6. Describe the use of chest X-rays and CBCs in diagnosing bacterial and viral infections.
7. Identify the clinical symptoms and treatment of pneumonia caused by bacterial infection.
8. Explain the clinical uses, mechanism of action, and antimicrobial spectrum of antibiotics used in treating bacterial pneumonia.
9. Discuss strategies for managing vaccine hesitancy among caregivers.

10.4.3 Case 3 Discussion

When addressing vaccine hesitancy, the healthcare provider should first listen to the caregiver's concerns and validate their feelings. The provider should then provide clear, evidence-based information about the benefits and risks of vaccination, avoiding medical jargon. It is important to check for understanding by asking the caregiver to summarize the discussion. Finally, the provider should reiterate the key points and ensure the caregiver feels supported in making an informed decision.

In this case, after the initial vaccine conversation, the child is admitted to the hospital due to a serious complication secondary to pertussis. Learners should discuss the importance of revisiting the vaccine conversation with the caregiver after such complications to reinforce the benefits of vaccination. This follow-up is crucial as it can help caregivers understand the real-world implications of vaccine-preventable diseases and may encourage them to reconsider their stance on vaccinations, ultimately protecting the health of their child and the community.

10.5 Case 4: Measles

This case focuses on the clinical features, pathogenesis, and prevention of a vaccine-preventable viral infection. Clinicians play a fundamental role in communicating with patients about vaccines and are typically their patients' primary source for vaccine information. Therefore, understanding the benefits of vaccination is crucial for health professions learners. Some vaccine-hesitant individuals believe that there is little risk to becoming infected with a vaccine-preventable infection. In this case, the child becomes susceptible to a life-threatening secondary bacterial infection.

10.5.1 Case 4 Clinical Vignette

Emily Johnson, a 4-year-old female, presents to her pediatrician, Dr. Lee, with a high fever, cough, runny nose, and conjunctivitis of 3 days duration. Mrs. Johnson indicates that Emily developed a rash starting on her face and spreading to her trunk and limbs over the past 24 h.

Physical Examination

Vitals: 39.5 °C (103.1 °F); HR 140; BP 90/55; RR 24; SpO2 95% on room air.

General: Alert but irritable. Well nourished; in no acute distress.

HEENT: PERRL. Red, watery eyes. Mild pharyngeal erythema without exudates. TMs clear.

Neck: A few scattered, nontender lymph nodes are palpable in the anterior cervical chains.

Integument: Erythematous maculopapular rash starting on the face and spreading to the trunk and limbs. Koplik spots noted on the buccal mucosa.

Dr. Lee informs Mrs. Johnson that Emily has measles. Dr. Lee inquires with Mrs. Johnson about Emily's measles, mumps, and rubella (MMR) vaccination status, and Mrs. Johnson indicates that she is opposed to vaccinations for health safety concerns. Neither Emily nor her older sister (age 6) have received the MMR vaccine. Mrs. Johnson asks Dr. Lee about the likelihood of other members of the family developing measles. Dr. Lee describes the mode of measles transmission and offers information on the benefits and risks of vaccination. She advises Mrs. Johnson to keep Emily out of school until at least four days after the onset of the rash.

Five days later, Emily returns to the clinic with a persistent high fever and difficulty breathing.

Physical Examination

Vitals: 40 °C (104 °F); HR 150; BP 85/50; RR 30; SpO2 92% on room air.

General: Crying and irritable.

HEENT: PERRL. Red, watery eyes. No pharyngeal or tonsillar erythema. TMs clear.

Neck: No lymphadenopathy.
Integument: Diffusely erythematous maculopapular rash.
Respiratory: Crackles heard in both lung fields.

Dr. Lee diagnoses Emily with measles-associated pneumonia and admits her to the hospital. A CBC with differential and chest X-ray are ordered. The chest X-ray shows bilateral infiltrates consistent with pneumonia. The peripheral white blood cell count is 18,000/mm^3 (reference = 4000–10,000/mm^3) with 85% neutrophils (reference = 40–80%).

Emily is diagnosed with bacterial pneumonia secondary to measles infection. She receives IV antibiotics with substantial improvement in her respiratory symptoms noted overnight. The following morning, IV antibiotics are changed to oral antibiotics, and Emily is discharged home.

Two days later, Dr. Lee phones Mrs. Johnson to inquire about Emily's status. Mrs. Johnson states that Emily's breathing has improved remarkably; however, she is concerned because her elderly mother is coming to visit. She asks Dr. Lee if she should notify her mother to cancel her trip because of Emily's measles. Dr. Lee states that her mother should avoid visiting until Emily has fully recovered, as measles can be particularly severe in older adults.

10.5.2 Case 4 Learning Objectives

1. Recognize the importance of childhood vaccine risk/benefit communication.
2. Describe the clinical presentation and complications of measles.
3. Describe the mode of transmission and course of infection of the measles virus.
4. Discuss the indications, contraindications, and formulation of the MMR vaccine.
5. Characterize the pathogenesis, diagnosis, and management of measles.
6. Describe how chest X-rays and CBCs are used in the diagnosis of bacterial and viral infections.
7. Describe the clinical symptoms and treatment of pneumonia caused by secondary bacterial infection.
8. Characterize the clinical uses, mechanism of action, and antimicrobial spectrum of antibiotics used in the treatment of bacterial pneumonia.
9. Differentiate between measles and other viral exanthems.

10.5.3 Case 4 Discussion

When addressing vaccine concerns, healthcare providers should follow a structured approach to ensure effective communication and understanding. Here's a detailed discussion framework:

1. *Elicit Concerns:* Begin by asking the patient or caregiver about their specific concerns regarding vaccination. This helps in understanding their perspective and addressing their fears directly.
2. *Label and Reflect Feelings:* Accurately label the emotions expressed by the patient or caregiver and reflect their intensity. For example, if a caregiver is anxious about vaccine safety, acknowledge their anxiety and validate their feelings.
3. *Provide Information:* Discuss the benefits of vaccination and the potential risks, using clear and simple language. Avoid medical jargon to ensure the information is accessible. Highlight the effectiveness of the MMR vaccine in preventing measles and its complications.
4. *Check for Understanding:* Ask the patient or caregiver to restate their understanding of the information provided. This step ensures that they have correctly understood the benefits and risks of vaccination.
5. *Summarize and Verify:* Conclude the discussion by summarizing the main points and seeking verification of understanding. This reinforces the key messages and ensures that the patient or caregiver is clear about the information shared.
6. *Revisit the Conversation:* In cases where complications arise, such as Emily's hospitalization due to bacterial pneumonia secondary to measles, it is beneficial to revisit the vaccine conversation. This provides an opportunity to reinforce the importance of vaccination in preventing such severe outcomes.

In this case, after Emily's hospitalization, Dr. Lee should circle back to the vaccine discussion with Mrs. Johnson. This follow-up conversation can help address any lingering doubts and emphasize the critical role of vaccines in protecting against serious diseases. By revisiting the topic, Dr. Lee can provide additional support and information, potentially influencing Mrs. Johnson's future decisions regarding vaccination for her children.

10.6 Case 5: Polio

This case focuses on the clinical features, pathogenesis, and prevention of polio, a vaccine-preventable viral infection. Clinicians play a fundamental role in communicating with patients about vaccines and are typically their patients' primary source for vaccine information. Therefore, understanding the benefits of vaccination is crucial for health professions learners. Some vaccine-hesitant individuals believe that there is little risk to becoming infected with a vaccine-preventable infection. In this case, the child becomes susceptible to a life-threatening condition due to lack of vaccination.

Polio, once a leading cause of paralysis among children worldwide, is very close to being eradicated. Since the establishment of the Global Polio Eradication Initiative (GPEI) in 1988, wild poliovirus types 2 and 3 have been eradicated, and global cases of wild poliovirus type 1 (WPV1) have decreased by over 99%. However, WPV1 remains endemic in Afghanistan and Pakistan. Additionally, outbreaks of circulating vaccine-derived poliovirus (cVDPV) continue to occur in underimmunized populations. Renewed efforts to vaccinate persistently missed children and strengthen routine immunization programs are essential to achieving global eradication.

10.6.1 Case 5 Clinical Vignette

Patient Information

Name: Ahmed Khan.

Age: 6 months.

Presenting to: Pediatrician, Dr. Johnson.

History: Ahmed Khan, a 6-month-old male, recently moved to the United States with his family from Pakistan, a country where polio has not been fully eradicated. Ahmed's parents, Mr. and Mrs. Khan, are concerned because Ahmed has developed a fever and weakness in his legs over the past two days. They mention that Ahmed has not received any vaccinations due to their concerns about vaccine safety.

Physical Examination

Vitals: 38.5 °C (101.3 °F); HR: 140; BP: 90/60; RR: 24; SpO2: 98% on room air.

General: Alert but irritable. Well-nourished; in no acute distress.

HEENT: PERRL. White sclerae. Mild pharyngeal erythema without exudates. TMs clear.

Neck: No lymphadenopathy.

Integument: No rashes or lesions.

Neurological: Decreased muscle tone in both legs. Reflexes diminished in lower extremities. No signs of meningeal irritation.

Dr. Johnson suspects poliomyelitis and inquires about Ahmed's vaccination status. Mrs. Khan expresses her concerns about vaccine safety and indicates that Ahmed has not received the polio vaccine. Dr. Johnson explains the importance of vaccination and the risks associated with polio, including paralysis and potentially life-threatening complications.

Laboratory Tests

CBC: WBC count within normal limits.

CSF Analysis: Elevated protein, normal glucose, and pleocytosis.

Stool Sample: Positive for poliovirus.

Diagnosis: Ahmed is diagnosed with acute flaccid paralysis due to poliovirus infection.

Management: Ahmed is admitted to the hospital for supportive care, including hydration, pain management, and physical therapy to prevent contractures and improve muscle strength. Dr. Johnson discusses the importance of vaccination with the Khans and provides information on the polio vaccine's safety and efficacy.

Follow-Up: Two weeks later, Ahmed shows some improvement in muscle strength but still requires ongoing physical therapy. Dr. Johnson continues to educate the Khans about the benefits of vaccination and encourages them to complete Ahmed's vaccination schedule to protect him from other preventable diseases.

10.6.2 Case 5 Learning Objectives

1. Recognize the importance of childhood vaccine risk/benefit communication.
2. Describe the clinical presentation and complications of poliomyelitis.
3. Describe the mode of transmission and course of infection of poliovirus.
4. Discuss the indications, contraindications, and formulation of the polio vaccine.
5. Characterize the pathogenesis, diagnosis, and management of poliovirus infection.
6. Describe the clinical symptoms and treatment of acute flaccid paralysis.
7. Discuss the global efforts and challenges in eradicating polio.

10.6.3 Case 5 Discussion

Following elicitation of the patient's or caregiver's chief concerns surrounding vaccination, the healthcare provider should accurately label their feeling and reflect its intensity. For example, Dr. Johnson might say, "I understand that you are worried about the safety of vaccines, and it's important to address these concerns."

Next, the provider should discuss the benefits of vaccination and potential risks while avoiding medical jargon. Dr. Johnson could explain, "Vaccines, including the polio vaccine, have been extensively studied and monitored for safety. The benefits of vaccinating Ahmed far outweigh the risks. Polio can cause severe paralysis and even be life-threatening, but the vaccine can protect him from these dangers."

The provider should check for understanding by asking the patient or caregiver to restate their understanding of the discussion. Dr. Johnson might ask, "Can you tell me what you understand about the benefits and risks of the polio vaccine?"

Finally, closure should be provided by briefly rephrasing the main points introduced in the discussion and seeking verification of understanding. Dr. Johnson could conclude, "To summarize, vaccinating Ahmed can protect him from serious diseases like polio. It's important to complete his vaccination schedule to ensure his health and safety. Do you have any other questions or concerns?"

In this case, after the provider has the vaccine conversation with the parents, the child is admitted to the hospital due to a dangerous condition caused by poliovirus. Learners should discuss the benefits of circling back to the vaccine conversation with the parents following the complication. This approach reinforces the importance of vaccination and addresses any lingering concerns the parents may have.

10.7 Conclusion

The five cases in this chapter provide a comprehensive framework for active-learning discussions on the importance of vaccination. Through real-life clinical scenarios, learners can explore the severe consequences of vaccine-preventable diseases and the essential role of healthcare providers in promoting vaccination. By facilitating these discussions, the cases aim to equip health professions learners with the skills needed to address vaccine hesitancy, communicate effectively with patients, and advocate for public health. These cases not only highlight the critical impact of vaccines but also reinforce the importance of informed, empathetic communication in clinical practice.

References

1. Makoul G. Essential elements of communication in medical encounters: the Kalamazoo consensus statement. Acad Med. 2001;76(4):390–3.
2. Centers for Disease Control and Prevention. Vaccine excipient summary. https://www.cdc.gov/vaccines/pubs/pinkbook/downloads/appendices/b/excipient-table-2.pdf
3. Centers for Disease Control and Prevention. Thimerosal and Vaccines. https://www.cdc.gov/vaccine-safety/about/thimerosal.html
4. Chase AJ, Clark MA, Rogalska A, Musselman M. Cultivating patient-physician communication about vaccination through vaccine metaphors. Med Sci Educ. 2020;30:1015–7. https://doi.org/10.1007/s40670-020-00981-6.
5. Scherer AM, Scherer LD, Fagerlin A. Getting ahead of illness: using metaphors to influence medical decision making. Med Decis Mak. 2015;35(1):37–45. https://doi.org/10.1177/0272989X14522547.

Index

A. J. Chase et al. (eds.), *Vaccine Hesitancy Curriculum*,
https://doi.org/10.1007/978-3-031-88668-3

MIX
Papier aus verantwortungsvollen Quellen
Paper from responsible sources
FSC® C105338

If you have any concerns about our products,
you can contact us on
ProductSafety@springernature.com

In case Publisher is established outside the EU,
the EU authorized representative is:
Springer Nature Customer Service Center GmbH
Europaplatz 3, 69115 Heidelberg, Germany

Printed by Libri Plureos GmbH
in Hamburg, Germany